THE TAOIST WAYS OF HEALING

A comprehensive introduction to the ancient Chinese health arts, the 'Eight Strands of the Brocade', as well as traditional techniques of diagnosis and 'The Way of Occlusion' — the overall method for achieving and maintaining perfect health, inner harmony and optimum internal and external energy at all levels.

GW00503645

THE
TAOIST WAYS
OF HEALING
The Chinese Art of Pa Chin Hsien

by

CHEE SOO

AQUARIAN

THE AQUARIAN PRESS
Wellingborough, Northamptonshire

First published 1986

British Library Cataloguing in Publication Data

Soo, Chee
   The Taoist ways of healing.
   1. Hygiene, Taoist
   I. Title
   610'.951   RA776.5

   ISBN 0-85030-475-X

*The Aquarian Press is part of the
Thorsons Publishing Group*

Printed and bound in Great Britain

Contents

Preface

From a Chinese point of view, it is very pleasing to know that more and more people in the West are taking a much greater interest in the ancient cultural arts of China, and are coming to understand the ways of Chinese thought, and how it can be adapted to day-to-day living in modern times. In this way they are beginning to appreciate the basic philosophy that is the very foundation of the entire Chinese nation, and of all those Chinese who live in other parts of the world, a philosophy that has been inbred into every thought and deed for thousands of years.

However, to appreciate fully every aspect of Chinese life and thought, the average person in the West will have to get rid of one very bad habit. Westerners tend to look at an object, or a symptom, or even a sentence, and immediately believe in what they see, read or hear, and accept it as it is presented to them. For instance, a Western doctor will see a wart on the skin, and try to reduce its size, or else will endeavour to remove it altogether by the use of surgery. Now the Chinese practitioner would tackle this problem in a completely different way — by trying to find what caused the wart to appear in the first place. He would then set about erasing the cause, and the symptom would eventually disappear, and no more symptoms would arise. If the problem is approached in the Western way, then there is no guarantee that the wart will not appear on another day.

Then there is the Western habit of taking a pill for a headache, which is another typical example of tackling the symptom rather than going direct to the cause. In this case the cause is the large intestine or the bladder, and so by eliminating the cause, which is coming from either of these organs, the sufferer ensures not only that the headache will disappear within a few seconds, but that there will be no reoccurrence of the trouble. That is the reason why the Chinese can get rid of migraines, once and for all, within twenty-four hours, without having to take a pill or medicine of any kind.

So this simple principle applies to all who have a sincere interest in China and all that it stands for, its deep-rooted culture and its philosophy. To turn this interest into understanding, you will have to look at China's past. In fact, you will have to go back some 12,000 years. Then, and only then, will you get to the true root of the matter, and develop an understanding that will be deep and lasting. Remember, if you want to appreciate what keeps a building standing upright for many centuries, have a close look at its foundations; there you will find the answer.

By going back in time, you will fully appreciate that the nature of the Chinese has been engrained with the philosophy, the culture and the knowledge that have been put there by thousands of years of deep education and understanding of the basic ways of living in accordance with the infinite laws of the universe. That everything in life must have its own unique balance, constantly maintaining harmony with everything around it, is one of the basic laws. Nothing can exist on its own, for all things link together to make the universe what it is — simply, one vast entity. To upset the delicate mechanism that creates and upholds the simple principles of nature is fatal, for it can lead to very serious repercussions in the form of stress, strife, wars and sickness in nature and within mankind.

Taoism has existed in China for at least 12,000 years. In fact the principles on which it is based were laid down thousands of years before that, although in that earlier period they were never given a specific name. To Chinese people at that time, these principles were simply a way of life that meant abiding by the infinite law of the universe as they knew it. By their simple attitudes to life, and their way of living from day to day, they gave the Chinese nation as a whole an ingrained philosophy which required no spoken words, and it therefore became an automatic lifeline which was passed down from one generation to the next.

It was the Taoists who kept alive many of the ancient arts and practices over the centuries, and they in turn gave greater understanding to the principles by which they lived, together with a full appreciation of everything that plays a part within the cosmos. They bridged the gap between heaven and earth, and thereby altered the mental outlook on, and attitudes to, the spiritual and the physical. In so doing, they found the 'Tao', the primeval law that regulates all matters within the universe, and recognized it as the Supreme Ultimate in all things.

It was this recognition that gave them the Yin and Yang, the two sides of everything, and it was this deep appreciation that completely altered their attitudes to everything that happened in their daily lives. It gave them the serenity of *acceptance,* and through this influence they were able to recognize the 'Tao' in everything.

Introduction

Outside of China very little is known of the vast range of therapeutic methods that have been studied and used for thousands of years on the Chinese mainland and are still being practised daily by Chinese everywhere in the world. But out of all the many sciences known to the Chinese, only one so far seems to have attracted the attention of the Western world, and that is acupuncture, and even the results that this art obtains are doubted by many medical professionals outside of China.

However, the vast wealth of experience has not gone entirely unnoticed, for Japan now uses traditional Chinese medical methods on an extensive scale, and the Academy of Sciences in the Soviet Union also has a department which has been making a special study of the Chinese methods and skills, and even in France and in Germany greater interest is being aroused through the medium of regular publications. In Britain, in addition to the Acupuncture Association, there are regular classes being held in London and elsewhere. Throughout Europe, too, there are various centres teaching the many arts of Chinese healing which together comprise Pa Chin Hsien (The Eight Strands of the Brocade). They all come under the auspices of the Chinese Cultural Arts Association and the International Taoist Society.

Why have the Chinese accomplished such advances in the understanding of the human body, while Western medical science, with all its vast resources, has still not been able to find the cures for such simple illnesses as sinusitis, migraine, arthritis, heart disease, varicose veins, bad nerves, sclerosis and many others? Millions of pounds and dollars are being squandered every year in the endeavour to find cures to the symptoms of illnesses, and yet in China, we have known the answers to all these illnesses, and have been able to understand the multitude of questions that are asked every day, for many thousands of years. In fact, even the common cold can be cured within forty-eight hours by the simple pressure of one finger, and migraine can be stopped just as suddenly in the same period through a simple dietary alteration. We seriously wonder how many millions of pounds and dollars have been wasted in fruitless attempts to find a pill that could do the same thing.

Beginnings: the 'Sons of Reflected Light' and the Early Taoists
How did the Chinese health arts begin? This is how my illustrious master, Professor Chan Kam Lee, told it to me in 1934: that some 12,000 years ago (approximately 10,000 BC), there arrived in China a race of people who were very tall indeed — reputedly over seven feet in height; and because of their unusual clothing they came to be known as the 'Sons of Reflected Light' (Fankuang Tzu). Where they came from is still a mystery, and perhaps the true answer to this question may never be known, but on their arrival they wasted no time, for they soon began to collect together a group of skilled people from many trades and professions, whose intelligence was above the normal average during that period.

Having collected this band of people together, they then began to instruct them in many different arts and crafts which technically were far in advance of anything that existed in those far-off days, and many of which have still not been bettered even to this present day.

It took many, many years to instruct the Chinese in the numerous sciences that in those early days were absolutely unheard of. Not only were they new but in many cases they were completely at odds with the Chinese way of life, and with their thinking at that time. Many died trying to learn all that was being taught to them. So it happened that their children, and in turn their children's children, had to carry on the work and the studies of these various arts.

They were taught many arts, including silk weaving, pottery making, the utilization of metals, and making and using gunpowder, making glass, and the most important of all, the vast range of health arts, such as herbal therapy, health diets, hot and cold treatments, massage, acupressure (spot pressing), respiration therapy and energy therapy.

Generation after generation have tried to carry on the work that these wonderful people bestowed upon mankind. Whether the

Chinese people have succeeded in remaining true to the original teachings, over the many centuries that have passed, only time will tell. It cannot be denied, however, that there is at least a possibility that during the many years that have gone by, and owing to the absence of early written records, some of those teachings have been lost.

After many centuries the 'Sons of Reflected Light' disappeared, and nothing seems to have been heard of them since, except that the foundations that they laid in all the years of their work have been built on through the years. Many of the family groups slowly dispersed throughout the length and breadth of China, and because of this, you will find that certain of the health arts became prominent in particular areas of the vast territory of China, mainly owing to the simple fact that some of the arts were more suitable to the local climate and natural environment of particular territories.

The impositions of some of the warlords and emperors in various districts also had some effect on the particular health arts that were practised there, and variations in philosophical and religious outlook also had a great bearing on the particular arts practised.

So it came to pass that whilst the health arts were taught in one place for many centuries, they eventually dispersed all over China, and local traditions were slowly built up around them. But it was the Taoists who brought them all back together again, so that their advancement in knowledge and skill was no longer hindered by local differences. The health arts blossomed anew under the philosophical guidance of the Taoists and through their aims of a healthy long life therapy for the body, their experimentation with the various channels of the mind, and their constant search for the growth, development and alchemy of the spirit. All this was made possible by the Taoists' simple understanding and knowledge of the energies that exist within ourselves and also that which is supplied by the universe.

Very early Taoist writings only began to appear in about 3000 BC, and one of the earliest was *The Yellow Emperor's Classic of Internal Medicine*, which is known as the *Nei Ching*, and many translations of this work have appeared in English, German and French. It comprises eighty-one chapters and is divided into two main sections, the Su Wen and the Ling Shu. The first part covers questions relating to the whole range of medical knowledge, while the second part deals with the spiritual essentials underlying medical treatment.

The Present Day — and Beyond

The health arts that the 'Sons of Reflected Light' (Fankuang Tzu) brought to China eventually came to be known as the 'Eight Strands of the Brocade' (Pa Chin Hsien), and even to this day, after thousands of years have passed, they are still known to the Chinese by that name. In the West these same arts are being used for the benefit of all those who wish to avail themselves of them, and in London there is a health clinic where these arts are used to help sufferers of all types of disease and infirmity, and it is completely free of charge.

Today, many young Chinese think that the 'Eight Strands of the Brocade' are merely a number of specialized breathing exercises, whereas the name properly refers to the complete Chinese Taoist health arts. The vast majority of people are completely unaware of the wide range that these arts cover, and even just how many of them there are. One of the more specialized sections, and one of the most well-known is acupuncture (Hsia Chen Pien), which along with all the other arts is still being carried on by many dedicated Chinese, both inside and outside of China. Since the Revolution, China has come to enjoy the best of two worlds, the very old and the new, and the ancient inheritance has been studied with greater enthusiasm than ever before. Together with modern Western medical science, which has since been introduced, the Chinese now have the best of three worlds.

The 'Eight Strands of the Brocade' (Pa Chin Hsien) actually comprise eight distinct health arts, and these are:

1. Ch'ang Ming (natural health dietary therapy).
2. Ts'ao Yao (herbal therapy).
3. Wen Chiech'u (thermology, or thermogenesis).
4. T'ui-Na or Anmo (Taoist massage).
5. Hsia Chen Pien (acupuncture).
6. Tien Chen (acupressure/spot pressing).
7. T'i Yu (physical calisthenics).
8. Ch'ili Nung (the Way of Occlusion).

In addition to the above there is also the utilization of the five senses, which are used for accurate diagnosis, but because it is not a specific healing art, it was never included in the list. However, everyone who studies our arts automatically learns to diagnose, both internally and externally, right from the very start, for it is the one sure way of finding out the true cause of an illness — rather than letting the symptom affect the judgement.

Many people wonder what kind of impact the Chinese health arts will have upon the medical profession in the West, and this we will have to see, but if they are willing to keep an entirely open mind in all they see and hear, and are willing to adapt their trends of thought to the Chinese ways of thinking, then they will encounter no problems at all.

In China, the patient and his welfare will always come first, for we are all of the same race (simply, the human race), and are therefore brothers and sisters, and if you should happen to lose one or the other, then it is completely natural for the whole family to be affected. Therefore in the Chinese medical profession, if it is considered that natural health therapy (Ch'ang Ming) or acupuncture (Hsia Chen Pien) can give quick and lasting results, then these will naturally be given first preference. Modern surgery will only be used as a very last resort, and not just as another means to an end, for practitioners of the Chinese health arts know that once you cut through nerves, blood vessels, skin tissue and bone, whilst these may recover in time, they are never completely the same as nature made them. Any form of surgery is therefore always considered to be the *very last resort.*

If the West were to adopt these same priorities then the patient would obtain the best from all fields of medical research, both old and new, but if Western medical professionals retain a closed mind and a closed shop to other forms of healing, then they will severely handicap themselves, since they will be limited to the only two methods of treatment on which they currently depend — namely, drugs and surgery. Drugs are made by big commercial companies, on whose research the doctors have to rely entirely. As for surgery, this is practised by a small minority group of medical specialists. Take these two away, and what has the modern doctor got left to offer his patients? Precisely nothing.

All healing arts should complement one another, for all things in the universe are in harmony with one another. The healing arts should also work in harmony, helping one another, seeking advice from each other, so that the whole of humanity can reap the benefits of the experience and knowledge of all fields. Good health is not the prerogative of one section of humanity; it should be available to all.

The great wealth of knowledge and practical experience that was built up over thousands of years has not gone to waste, but is alive, and available to all mankind. The Western world, whose medicine has a history of less than two hundred years, would do well to take a little more interest in these arts that have been proved over and over again through thousands of years.

It is like comparing the growth of an ant to that of an elephant. A child should not be jealous of an adult, for he too can learn everything that the adult has learned, or more, providing that he is willing to study hard and diligently. The adult, in turn, should not look down on the ignorance of the child, for the adult was once an infant himself. That is why the Chinese are always willing to pass on their knowledge to all, whether they are just ordinary human beings or fully qualified scientists, providing they are all willing to learn as much as they can, and yet at the same time keep a completely open mind.

To all those who have suffered every day of their lives, and there may be more who have been in agony for many years, and have tried every known treatment in the West, including every conceivable drug, then it will be truly worthwhile to let the Chinese demonstrate what they can do.

You will be amazed at the results that can be obtained, but you will have to be dedicated in your effort to be cured, once and for all time, if you want to gain the supreme benefits that the Chinese Taoist health arts can offer.

Chapter 1

The Tao

The Taoist does not have to put a name to his consciousness of the workings of the Supreme Spirit, nor to his awareness that this work is going on around him every day of his life, nor to the principles by which all nature is ordered. Thus he learns to abide by the infinite laws of the universe which govern all things, past, present and future.

Most people consider the Taoist to be a mystic, just because he does not build images to worship, hang pictures on the wall to remind him of his faith, or put another human being on a pedestal and worship him. On this last point, the Taoist believes that even the greatest of humans can never be more than a sage or a philosopher, spreading his understanding through word of mouth or through the medium of his writings.

The Taoist has no rituals, no altars, and no expensive ceremonial garments, for he lives with his maker every day of his life, and strives to conquer his innermost self so that one day he may be proved worthy to help and assist others in their struggle to find the true Way of their own life, and thereby fully appreciate the true meaning of the Tao.

But, you might well ask, what is the Tao? Well! This is the simplest question to answer, for here it is:

It is as simple as that, and isn't that easy? It is nothing within nothing, yet it comprises all things inside and outside; it is the sole controller of everything that lives and grows; it is the energy that creates and gives life to all things, including ourselves; it is the destiny that governs every incident that occurs, and even those that do not. It is the strength and weakness of every element, it is the good and the bad, for truly speaking there is neither. It is the happiness and sadness that pervades our emotions; it is the spiritual and the physical; it is the monolithic duality of all things. It is the Yin and the Yang. It is simply the ordained Way of every single individual, and of every single plant, bush, tree and animal, as well as the formation of the clouds, the rainfall, the ice and snow, and also the sunshine — it is indeed the Tao of all and of everything.

That is why there can be no name for it, nor any definition; for it cannot be seen, and only its work and the results it obtains are visible to human eyes, providing that you keep your eyes open all the time, and allow the results of what you see to register in your mind. It is older than the universe, yet younger than something that is born at this very moment in time. It is not something within something, yet it is the influence or guiding principle of the Tao that makes things what they are, and what they are to be. It is not destiny or fate, for the Tao created them too. It is not energy, yet it is the infinite laws of Tao behind and within it. It is, in its simplest definition, the will of the Supreme Spirit, or God, if you want to use that name.

So those who call the Taoist a mystic have no appreciation or understanding of the workings of the universe, nor do they comprehend the balance that is created and exists within all things, Even more so, they are not religious in any way, for they do not understand the work of their own God.

The Tao cannot be bought, possessed, transmitted or heard, yet it can be seen as clearly as you read the words on this page, and I hope to give you some examples so that you can begin to open your eyes, instead of living your daily life completely blind to the workings of the Tao (the Supreme Spirit — Yuang Tati). Everyone can find the truth of the Tao within himself, providing that he keeps a completely open mind, and does not allow any thoughts to invade the privacy of his brain, nor any emotions to block the channels to his own spirit.

The first step is to get rid of all words, and stop trying to put everything into different categories or individual filing cabinets. Don't bracket everything as good or bad; learn to accept it as being ordained, for there is no such thing as good luck, good fortune, a lucky break, or a wonderful coincidence; and neither is there such a thing as misfortune, an unlucky coincidence or a stroke of bad luck. It was ordained to be, for it is the will of the Tao, so learn to accept it as a part of your life and your true destiny here on this earth. After all, you accept that day will follow night, and night will follow day, and you don't jump with joy just because it happens, and neither do you go into hysteria or the depths of despondency just because you wanted daylight and it happens to be pitch black at midnight. No, you accept this daily phenomenon of the universe as completely normal and natural, yet it is the Tao that made and controls this simple daily routine, and you accept it every day of your life without any query or emotion.

Rain follows sunshine, sunshine follows rain, and whilst you might curse a wet or windy day, especially if you are all dressed up to go somewhere special, you do not query the fact that it happens; you learn to accept it as an infinite part of nature, so once again you have accepted it as the will of the Tao.

You put a seedling into the garden and watch it grow into a beautiful plant. In so doing you have accepted its growth as completely natural, just as much as you accept the weeds that will grow around your seedling that you had planted. So be it, the will of the Supreme Spirit (Tao) has shown you the natural Way of your plant but also the ordained destiny of the weeds that grew around it, and you cannot alter the rules of their growth, for these have been laid down since the very beginning of time.

All right, you accept the growth and natural movements of nature and of the universe, and the many changes that go on within them, but you will, no doubt, still ask how the Tao comes into your own life, and how it affects you personally.

This is very simply answered. First it was ordained in what period of time you should be born, then what country you should be born in, and it is not by chance that you happened to be born in the British Isles, or the United States of America, or in Australia, for you could have been born in Africa, China or South America if it had been the will of the Tao. Next, who will be your parents, should they be rich or poor, will they live to be very old so that you will have them near you for a very long time, or will you lose them in your early life, to give you greater internal strength from having to stand on your own feet much earlier in life? What schools will you go to, what kind of work will you do — preacher, carpenter, pilot, business executive —? Long before you were born, all these things were planned by the will of the Tao.

How many times in the past have you chased different jobs when you were out of work, only to find that they had all gone? And then, perhaps, one that you least expected to get, or for which you seemed least qualified, suddenly landed in your lap. If so, that was not luck or chance; it was ordained to be, for it was the work of your own Tao.

Have you ever been to a seaside town on a bank holiday expecting every car park to be full, and then been amazed to find an empty space already waiting for your arrival? Well, that was not luck or even a coincidence, for it had already been planned for you. It was a part of the Tao of your life, so say your prayers and thank the Supreme Spirit for arranging it for you.

Now this applies to every single person here on this earth, and it happens every single day of your life, in every place, in all you do, night and day, and all incidents will have their good aspects (Yang) and their periods of low ebbs (Yin). It is in the low ebb times that you will have the greatest feeling of stress, for this is how the cycle of time and motion works. It is in these patches that violence, emotional upsets, accidents and bad thoughts become more prevalent, and in certain portions of these periods you may also feel run down or extremely tired.

Therefore in these periods you will come up against situations that will need your innermost strength, for some things may happen without any apparent reason. Unbeknown to us, however, at the time there are reasons behind it, and you must learn to accept them as they come along, for they are still the will of the Tao.

All these things are tests for your spirit, and they pave the way for your greater inner strength, including your mental and spiritual spheres, and also your physical advancement, and you may see your innermost weaknesses if only you will give yourself sufficient time to look and appreciate each situation in its true light. Very few people in our modern society turn their eyes inwards and look at themselves at all, and even fewer look at and appreciate everything that happens in each second of their lives.

Therefore, if you should go under, by becoming emotionally upset, deeply depressed, losing your temper, resorting to violence, or just hating others for something that they have said or done, then you have definitely failed in the struggle to control yourself, and you have also failed to strengthen your mental and spiritual self. So you will be punished for your bad thoughts or deeds, for this an automatic retribution (Yin Kuo). But you will also get more and more tests in the future until you have proved that you are strong enough to get over that particular hurdle, and the others to come, and that you have developed the will to take everything in your stride as it comes along, with the same smile, the same calmness of attitude, and the same outlook on life — just as you have learnt to accept night and day, rain and sunshine, plants growing and dying, and the good times in your life.

That is what is meant by accepting the natural laws of the universe, because everything else which is made by man is completely artificial and superficial, and in other words, it is simply the difference between heaven and earth. Heaven is represented by the will of the Tao and the natural laws that it has laid down, whereas earth represents the commercial and unnatural laws that have been formulated by human beings.

Simplicity is the foundation of all the natural laws, and the Taoist sees and understands it, and within himself endeavours to live accordingly. Most human beings, however, do tend to make even the simplest things complicated, and they create greater misunderstanding by the use of too many words, when in actual fact no words are really necessary. If there doesn't happen to be a word to fit a particular situation or article, then they invent one. This applies to governments as well, for every day they sit and make more and more laws, so not only do they create further tension and stress amongst their fellow men, but they also greatly increase further intolerance and tension by upsetting the balance of normal and natural lives.

So by making an item more complicated than it should have been they now also create the opportunity for other people to make their own interpretations, and thereby it is made even more complicated than it was before. There is an old Taoist saying that goes back thousands of years: 'Man may create one improvement, but in so doing, he will also create one defect.' In other words, man may think that he is making an unqualified improvement, but in actual fact he automatically creates a defect. Why is this? The answer is that by trying to make an improvement, he has altered the balance of Yin and Yang, and therefore he will always get a reverse effect at the same time as the one intended. That is why you cannot upset the natural laws of the universe which were made by the Tao.

Now perhaps you are beginning to appreciate that it is an impossibility to describe the indescribable. How can it be possible to write or give a name to the will of the Supreme Spirit, for every blade of grass, every plant, every tree, every bird, every animal, and every human, has its own ordained way of life, and although two blades of grass might seem the same, they will still differ from one another, for they have their own individuality, exactly the same as humans, and therefore each will have its own span of life.

That is why the Taoists of China, in their infinite wisdom, knew that they could not give a different individualistic description to everything that exists. To cover the enormity of the task, and to describe the Will of the Supreme Spirit, they gave it the simplest of names — the Tao, which explains everything and yet, in its own typical Chinese way, describes nothing. Look inside it, or look at the other side of it, and also look into the depths of it, then eventually the true meaning will be made known to you, and then, and only then, you will find that you don't even need the word Tao to cover it, for as I have said earlier, it is truly indescribable. It has been like this since time immemorial, and even before the universe came into being, and it will remain so for the rest of eternity.

In the very beginning there was no universe, in fact there was literally nothing, for there was a void, and it was there that the Supreme Spirit (Yuhuang Tati) resided. It ordained that everything should have a balance of two sides, just like a coin, and this is what was described by the Taoists as the Yin and Yang. The energy that created everything was the energy of the Supreme Spirit, and we call this macrocosmic energy (Ching Sheng Li). It was this energy that was the first to abide by the rules and the duality of the Yin and Yang. It was because of this duality that the universe was created over five billion years ago. The human race is only five million years old, so there is an enormous difference.

Because the Supreme Spirit ordered that everything should conform to this duality, even the Ying and the Yang had to have two sides, plus a neutral zone between the two, which in total gave the five complete sections, which the Taoists named the 'Five elements' (Wu Hsing), and it was from these that all life became possible. It started off with vegetation, then the fishes, and then animal life, then finally the human race. That is how we all came into existence, and how we have remained here on this planet ever since.

Unless man learns to live in accordance with the basic rules of the Yin and Yang and the Five Elements, and learns also to follow the unwritten yet natural laws of the Supreme Spirit, then the human race will wither away and die. The deterioration has already set in, and more and more humans are now dying each and every year, for man is slowing killing man, not only through wars and other forms of violence, but by upsetting the basic law of the Tao, which is the Will of the Supreme Spirit.

Chapter 2

Yin and Yang

There is constant harmony and also opposition within everything in the universe, and this includes the human body. It is these opposing and unifying factors that are known as the two poles of the infinite, referred to by the Taoists of China as the Yin and Yang.

Yin signifies all things that are negative, contractive, cold, dark, thin and feminine, whereas Yang denotes the complete opposite, which is positive, expansive, hot, light, fat and masculine. But it should be remembered that all phenomena in the universe are constantly on the move, and therefore changing, and although the fluidity of the universe cannot always be seen, it is always in a state of flux. Remember that nothing is ever totally motionless, nor is it always in fast motion, and so whilst these fluctuations and changes take place, it must be appreciated that nothing is entirely Yin and also that nothing is completely Yang. Therefore all phenomena are naturally relative to one another.

Yin and Yang are the will of the Tao, so they represent the universal laws of heaven and earth; they are the governors of all living matter, mother and father of all change, masters of time and motion, and the originators of birth and death. *The Yellow Emperor's Classic of Internal Medicine*, known as the *Nei Ching*, states quite simply that 'Yin is active within and is the guardian of the Yang, whereas Yang is the dominant force on the outside and it is the regulator of the Yin' — therefore Yin will produce and protect Yang in the infinity, and Yang will provide and control Yin in the extremity.

It must be understood also that everything has its maximum and minimum levels. For instance, you can take either the Yin or the Yang up to its natural maximum level, but once having reached that point, then it will automatically revert back again. Try two examples of these explicit laws. First, throw a ball into the air, and secondly, try stretching a piece of elastic, and see what happens. So from this you will appreciate that Yin will turn Yang at some point or another, and the same procedure will apply to Yang, which will turn to Yin, but of course under different circumstances.

You can walk from the centre of a room outwards, but you can get only as far as the walls, then you have got to turn back if you want to keep your motion going. Exactly the same thing happens within nature. Here is another complex situation, for Yang is never totally Yang, for at certain levels or periods in time it will become Yin — and vice versa — and this normal reaction applies quite naturally to the health of the human body.

Yang illnesses can be cured by Yin treatment, and Yin sicknesses can be overcome by Yang influence, cancer being an example of the latter. Cancer is caused by the extreme influence of Yin and to get the sufferer back to a healthy state, you have to make that cancer change direction. By creating the circumstances, internally and externally, that will make it turn Yang, it can be beaten very easily, providing sufficient time is allowed.

Nothing is totally Yin and nothing is completely Yang, for they constantly interplay and interrelate with one another, and neither of them can exist entirely on its own, for their entire subsistence depends on their relationship to one another. For instance, just take a look at an ordinary cup, which is Yang. Its inside, however, is Yin. Now take the outer shell of it away, which is the Yang part, and what have you got left? Nothing. Now bring it back, and fill the centre of the cup with more clay, by making the void in the centre more Yang, and what have you got left? No cup. For a cup (Yang) is only a cup when you have a void (Yin) in the centre.

As we have mentioned before, these two rely entirely on one another and therefore it is necessary to harmonize, and yet both are in constant conflict, and therefore opposed. So it only needs a slight tipping of the scales to make either of them go one way or the other. An evenly balanced harmony between the two will mean good health, but even the slightest displacement in either direction could mean sickness.

So in terms of health and Chinese Taoist medicine, the interplay of Yin and Yang exerts its influence on the two energies of 'macrocosmic energy' (Ching Sheng Li), which is the energy of the universe, and 'internal energy' (Neichung Ch'i), which is the energy within the human body. Both of these can have a great influence on the good health of every individual, and that is why they are the roots of Chinese diagnosis and pathology.

Macrocosmic energy (Ching Sheng Li) is Yang when compared with internal energy (Neichung Ch'i), which is accepted as Yin in comparison, but both have within them the balance of the Yin and the Yang. For your further understanding, Li is the energy of the Supreme Spirit which it allowed out of the void and which formed the whole universe through the will of the Tao.

This energy originally swept out of the void and into the universe creating order from the chaos that existed at that time, and that is how the planetary systems came into being and how the earth on which we live was formed. The void, the home of the Supreme Spirit, is Yin, and the outward expansion of Li energy was therefore Yang, and it still maintains this balance and holds each planet in its pre-selected place, and it is also in continuous flow, even as you read this, and still enters into our earth every second of every day.

As Li energy comes into the earth's atmosphere it passes through all Yang things, before entering the soil, and once the world has been filled to its maximum capacity, then the overflow returns back to heaven (if you wish to call it that) from whence it came, and therefore it is now Yin, and it will now pass through all Yin things on its return journey back to its original home. The Yang direction of flow of Li energy looks something like this:

Naturally, as it moves further away from heaven, it becomes weaker, and as the spirit of man is Yang, this Li energy will naturally pass through the human body as well, by going down the spine and out through the abdomen, in a centripetal circular motion (as depicted above). It then continues its journey by going into the earth. It will naturally pass through other Yang things, such as Yang birds and animals, and also Yang vegetation, wood being one form of the latter.

Conversely, it also passes through all Yin things on its way back to 'heaven' and as women have Yin spirits, it will pass through them, in a centrifugal circular action, by rising up through the spince and out through the head. The Taoists represented this flow of direction like this:

When the Taoists put the two together, the result was the now very well-known Yin and Yang symbol, which everyone associates with China:

As we now know, this represents the direction of flow of Li energy in men and women, and in all Yang and Yin objects, and so it represents the unity and duality, the dual monism, in all things here on this earth.

Internal energy (Neichung Ch'i) is more commonly known as the 'vitality power' (Sheng Ch'i), and it refers to your own personal energy, for only you can cultivate, develop and control it. Whereas Li energy moves through the tissue and bone, Ch'i energy circulates through the body along the lines of the meridians, or energy channels. Li is absolutely necessary for the life of the spirit, and Ch'i is required for the support system of life within the human body, and both manifest themselves in entirely different ways.

Internal energy is the natural energy of the human body, and everyone is born with it. It is this natural power source that enables you to do your daily work, for it is the energy that gives life to all your organs, muscles and blood vessels. It also helps to revitalize the various functional, control and psychic centres within the body, so that they become not only more supple and more flexible but also more receptive. It therefore enables them to have a much larger scope for their work.

Internal energy also helps to fight off the attacks of bacteria that invade the human body, and so if you are truly healthy then you are never ill. One true and positive sign of the health of your own body is whether you ever catch a cold. If you do suffer from this malady every year, then you are definitely a sick person, for if you are truly healthy, then you never catch a cold at all, since the bacteria are killed off naturally by the strength and health of your internal energy. The Taoists of China have a saying: 'If you catch one cold in your lifetime then you are physically sick, and if you lose your temper once in a lifetime then you are mentally sick.'

If you are truly healthy, then you are automatically fit; but being fit does not necessarily mean that you are healthy: even athletes catch colds. So good health means that all the natural processes of the body, plus the strength of your internal energy, are in balance with one another and therefore in perfect harmony, and this is always being constantly maintained even though minute fluctuations and changes are always taking place within the whole system. Should imbalances or disturbances occur then it is natural for structural decay and malfunctions to take place, simply because of the lack or weakness in the internal energy which should have been strong enough to maintain a perfect equilibrium between all the factors involved.

So any disturbance of the proper balance within all things in the human body, will, if allowed to continue, tend to shorten the normal lifespan. Such an imbalance can be so minute that it may never be seen as an outward symptom, and so it can go undetected for years and years, and in some cases may never be known at all. In other cases where there is drastic disturbance, then the obvious signs can be very distressing not only to the person concerned, but also to the entire family.

This is where the Chinese Taoist art of Pulse Study (Chen Mo) has proved its worth a million times over, for nothing in the human body, internally or externally, can be hidden, and therefore, irrespective of the symptoms or lack of them, the cause is always known. For not only does it tell us the health of the body as a whole, but it can also tell us the history and the present story of each individual organ.

Before going into the study of Chen Mo let us now look at the Five Elements (Wu Hsing), which are so closely related to the Yin and Yang.

Chapter 3

The Five Elements

We now know that Yin and Yang are in intricate balance in all things within the universe, and also that they quite naturally manifest themselves, in varying degrees and proportions, according to the 'form'.

Having fully confirmed their observations concerning these two, the-ancients of China then realized that even Yin and Yang had within them a similar duality, which was simply the balance of change that takes place, for each one could ascend from a minimum point to a maximum level, or descend from the extreme to the lowest plane.

This can easily be seen in the growth of a plant, which first grows from a seed, rears itself to maturity, and then at its climax blossoms and shows the world its beauty before bearing its seed. Then the state of decline comes for it sheds its leaves, and then the plant itself falls to the ground, and the plant itself eventually dies, but in so doing it acts as a cover and a fertilizer for the seed, and then the plant rests during the cold winter months. The next year it goes through the same cycle of growth and decay.

So it was that the Taoists, appreciating that this cycle must also apply to everything in the cosmos, understood that such changes also occurred within themselves, and as such were closely linked to the fluctuations that existed within Yin and Yang. So they decided to split the principles of each into two, which gave them the Yin and Yang of each part, plus a neutral section in between, when they reached the stage of changing from one to the other. This then gave them five sections of change or cyclic vacillations, and because these gave life to nature, and nature in turn was able to make the ancients aware of these constant differentials, so it came about that the Taoists gave them the names of the five basic elements of nature.

These elements are fire, wood, earth, metal and water, and they can all complement each other in their work or oppose each other, and in sò doing cause their own deterioration. Fig. 1 shows how they harmonize wih each other. Each element gives way to the next. Wood is food for the fire, and when it turns to ashes then it naturally becomes a part of the earth, and from the earth comes metal, and metal in its molten state is like water, and water is nourishment for the trees, which gives us the wood, and thereby the circle is complete.

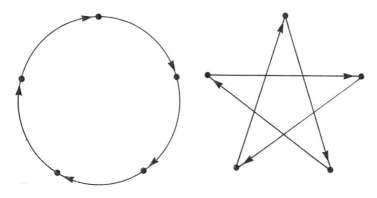

Fig. 1 The Harmony of the Five Elements.

However, because there is a balance of the duality within all things in the universe, these same elements can also oppose one another. For example, metal can chop down wood, wood in turn can draw the goodness from the earth, earth can absorb or dam the water,

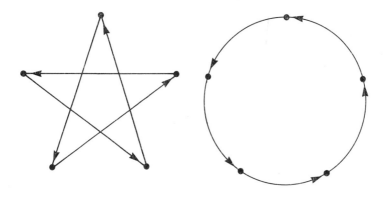

Fig. 2 The Opposition of the Five Elements.

water will put out the fire, and fire will make the metal melt. So each in turn can affect the efficiency of the others or even destroy them, depending on the particular situation and the law of relativity, which will decide whether the minimum or maximum level will apply to that condition. (See Fig. 2.)

From these base elements of the universe, as the ancient Chinese formulated them, grew plant life, then animal life, and then the human race. So all life forms are interrelated even though human beings have been slow to admit that they are animals.

The five elements, then, refer to everything in the universe. Hence we have groups of five, such as the five directions, the five colours, and the five 'naked-eye' planets, as well as the five Yin organs and five Yang organs of the human body. These organs are linked with the five elements as follows:

Elements	Yang Organs	Yin Organs
Fire	Small Intestine	Heart
Wood	Gall Bladder	Liver
Earth	Stomach	Spleen/Pancreas
Metal	Large Intestine	Lungs
Water	Urinary Bladder	Kidneys

The Yang organs were considered to be those that were related to function in connection with some influences outside of the body, whilst the Yin organs had a primary internal operation action and value. So it will be appreciated how closely linked the five elements are to the principles of the Yin and the Yang.

It is for this very reason that humanity must recognize that everyone in the world is very closely allied to nature, and is organically an integral part of the universe, and therefore is, and always will be, the fulfilment of the Tao.

Because humanity and nature are so closely linked, it was completely natural for the ancient Chinese Taoists to assume that each could have an influence on the other, in either a harmonious or an inharmonious role, and so it was that they began to use these same principles in their diagnosis, and in the vast range of their healing arts. So whilst the philosophy, understanding and practice of the Taoist healing arts began in the realms of antiquity, the modernist should not be under the impression that they are outmoded, for both the principles and the arts themselves are still being used today with enormous success and are attracting increasing interest from modern medical science.

Chapter 4

Traditional Diagnosis

The Five Elements

As the Five Elements are linked to the Yin and Yang, and these in turn are governed by the Tao, it is understandable that curing illness is also linked to the Five Elements. These cures are:

Fire	spiritual cure
Wood	Ch'ang Ming
Earth	herbal therapy
Metal	acupuncture
Water	thermogenesis

The Spiritual Cure

The spiritual cure comes about by altering your eating and drinking habits so that you become closer to nature, and thereby closer to your own Tao and the Supreme Spirit. In addition, it means becoming more understanding, more conscious, and more aware of the work of the Supreme Spirit that goes on around you, and learning to conform to the infinite laws that he has laid down. It means dedicating your life to helping others along the pathway of their lives, and in turn trying to make them understand as well. It also means that you should say your prayers in thanks for everything that is bestowed upon you, the food that you eat, the clothing that you wear, the car that you own, and every time you safely cross the road, or find a parking space. It is not luck that brings you home safely every evening, but the gift of the Supreme Spirit, so say 'thank you' a hundred times a day for all the gifts you receive.

Ch'ang Ming

Ch'ang Ming is the Taoist's natural eating and drinking system, and it will cure the majority of illnesses. It means eating good wholesome and natural foods, so carefully balanced that sickness is eradicted and ill health becomes a thing of the past. Remember that one of the most simple of all indicators of general sickness is the common cold. If you catch a cold every year, then you are in real trouble, and you have no one to blame but yourself, for you have created the cause that has brought about the symptom.

The food that you eat and the fluid that you drink must be within the boundaries of the universal laws and the very fine balance of Yin and Yang.

Herbal Therapy

Herbal therapy has long been a part of Chinese medical history, as it has also been with every other country in the world. But the Chinese have far exceeded the efforts of other nations in this particular field. With over 30,000 herbs on record they have found the answer to every conceivable illness, and according to the traditional classification, they have also listed them in order of the Yin and Yang tendencies.

Modern traditional herbal therapeutics have further divided these two groups into a further three sections under each heading, and have recorded them as either vegetable, animal or mineral. Naturally the vegetable section is the largest of the three.

Acupuncture

Acupuncture has been practised in China for thousands of years and is the simple insertion of a needle at a specific point or points along an energy channel, or meridian, as it is more commonly known. This will either stimulate or sedate the energy force that flows along that particular channel, which in turn has its links with a specific organ. Over nine different needles used to be available, varying in length and thickness, although in the beginning stone needles were in common use, and it was much later that copper and iron needles were used.

Thermogenesis

Thermogenesis is another ancient art of China. It works by combating an inner Yin illness with an external Yang force — applied heat. This Yang heat has two main objectives, either to draw the Yin cause to the surface by attraction, or to penetrate into the body and overcome or destroy the Yin in its own centre. For the best results, the heat is generally applied to the acupuncture points, and in the old days the skin was actually burned and many of the older Chinese still bear scars reminding them of their earlier treatment. Today, however, the skin is only warmed through, and no burning is necessary. There are, however, certain points along the lines of a meridian where heat treatment is absolutely banned or strictly forbidden, although acupuncture may be used.

Diagnosis

Whilst it is important to know how to effect a cure, it is even more essential to understand the cause, and traditional Chinese doctors are elevated in this particular field, utilizing the 'five methods of examination' (Wun Chen Ch'a):

1. Using the mouth to ask questions.
2. Using the eyes to see the symptoms and the indication of the possible causes.
3. Using touch, to feel lumps and to induce muscular reaction by light pressure. In addition touch was used in the art of Pulse Study (Chen No).
4. Using the ears to hear the changes of tone in the voice, as well as the percussions of the lungs, or the rumblings and other sounds in the bowel systems of the body.
5. Using the nose to smell the odours emanating from the various regions of the body, such as the mouth, sexual organs, anus, under the armpits, etc.

Asking Questions

Asking questions might seem quite an ordinary thing to do, but it is a very responsible job, and not always that easy to do with shy or reticent patients. However, it is necessary to fully understand the person's complaint, its development, how long it has gone on for, the person's eating and drinking habits, any accompanying aches or pains and how long they last, and whether it is painful at a specific time of the day. It is also sometimes useful to know the area of the world that they were born in, also the eating habits of the parents, and whether there are any hereditary tendencies in the family, and if so, how far back in time these inclinations seem to go.

It is also necessary to enquire about more personal things, such as the colour or smell of the urine, or the motions, regularity of periods and the types of pain that come with them, difficulties in intercourse, and any soreness in or around the other cavities of the body. A delicate approach is of course required for this questioning.

Naturally there are further difficulties when you have to interview young children, the mentally handicapped, or the deaf or the dumb. They will all have difficulty in explaining their particular illness, the type of pain, even how long they have had it, and as for remembering past symptoms this is almost an impossibility for those in the first two categories, so it will be necessary to obtain as much information as you can from their relatives or even close friends. When attempting to diagnose someone who is unconscious, you will of course have to rely entirely on background information from others.

All this information will give you the patient's general medical history so far as it relates to the complaint, as well as giving you an indication of the person's eating and drinking habits, which can have a very great influence on health. As you will see, asking questions is a very important part of the process of diagnosis.

Using the Eyes

Visual observation diagnosis is very important too, for it can supply extremely useful data on the present health of the person, and likely problems that may crop up in the future. In many cases you can also see if the illness has gone on for a long time. In other instances, you may be able to see the start of an illness, or detect the actual sickness, even though the person concerned does not have any outward symptoms, such as pains, rashes, vomiting, or hot or cold spells. It is quite possible that even the patient himself does not know that he is ill, so you will be able to combat the possible cause of the sickness even before the onset of symptoms.

Visual diagnosis is more important than many Westerners realize, for it means that the traditional doctor can examine parts of his patient without that person being aware that they are being inspected, or that an assessment of symptoms and the cause of illness has been mentally recorded.

First of all, the colour and texture of the skin on the face and hands will be immediately visible, and there may be many colours that can be seen, such as red, brown, white, yellow, grey, purple, semi-transparent white, and even green, and all these colours will indicate the general health of the person, and also show the possible cause of it. For instance a yellow skin is an outward sign of jaundice, which in turn indicates that there are problems with the pancreas, and possibly the liver and gall bladder as well. Red shows that the heart is overworking; very dark brown or black is associated with the kidneys; grey shows that the liver is swollen so trouble can be expected; white is generally anaemia; transparency in the skin shows either skin complaints or tuberculosis; and green, which is getting more and more common in the Western world, is cancer.

The general texture of the skin may be dry, oily or wet, and there may be excessive growth of hair. Dry skin shows skin complaints; oily skin is caused by overeating; wet skin indicates that the person drinks too much fluid, which in turn can affect the kidneys and may have a detrimental effect on the heart; and excessive hair, especially over the organs of the body, will show that a particular organ is under stress and is overworking.

Look at the fingernails: if there are white spots or flashes then this is a sure sign of excess consumption of sugar, sweets or fruit. There should be no half moons at the at the base of the nail; if they are present they indicate toxins in the bloodstream, and the bigger the half moons, the greater the problem. Long, thin nails are Yin whilst a short, broad nail is Yang. The natural grain of the nail should run from top to bottom. If the grains is deeply rutted or runs deeply across the nail, then it could show that there are bacteria in the intestine, or worms, and that there is a very erratic pattern of eating.

Now let us have a look at the face, which can supply us with a wealth of information. Vertical lines between the eyebrows indicate a bad liver, which will make the patient temperamental — so watch out. Erratic lines running across the forehead show a split personality, but evenly spaced parallel lines are a sign of excessive fluid consumption, so there could be an effect on the kidneys.

If the eyebrows are long and thick, this shows vitality, long life and happiness; if they are very thin this show Yin weaknesses; and if there is no eyebrow at all, cancer is indicated. The eyebrow should follow the natural curvature of the eye if you are Yang, but if you are Yin and the eyebrows turn upwards at the ends towards the temples, then it is a positive sign of weaknesses in the system, lack of vital energy, and that you have been eating too much meat for a very long time.

The eyelashes should be strong and straight but if they curl upwards then the person is Yin and it is a sign of bad health caused through the consumption of too much meat and meat products, and in a woman it shows that her ovaries are deeply contracted, so if she ever has a baby then the child is going to be affected by the same influence.

The eyes themselves have their own story to tell. Long, thin eyes with the iris centralized are a sign of good health. White large, round eyes denote susceptibility to colds and flu, for the general health is weak and very delicate. If both eyes turn outwards towards the ears, then there is far too much toxin in the body, and if the energy of the body is depleted to lower levels in the future, there is always the possibility of cancer showing its effects. On the other hand, crossed eyes is a sign of being too Yang and therefore there is a tendency towards high blood pressure. If the white of the eye can be seen not only on both sides of the iris but also above it as well, then the person is very Yin. Such people are cruel, will argue on the slightest pretext, and will lose their temper for no apparent reason, therefore being completely unpredictable.

If the white of the eye changes in colour, then this indicates a variety of Yin illnesses. Yellow is linked with jaundice, and red shows a liver complaint. Grey or blue means that the eyesight is declining, and if the symptom is ignored then blindness will eventually result. Coloured spots on the white of the eye near the iris denote also that there are various body malfunctions, and unless dietary improvements are made soon then the patient can expect serious internal trouble.

Bags under the eyes, if they are soft and spongy, signify that there is too much fluid in the body, in which case the kidneys will be overworking, but if the bags have a tendency to be firm or even hard, then this is a sure sign of the formation of kidney stones.

Always try to look at the edge of the bottom eyelid, for this is one place that make-up cannot hide. If it is white then the person is anaemic, and if it is red then there is inflammation due to infection and it has come to the surface as an outward symptom of excessive consumption of meat, sugar and fruit.

Discharge of fluid from the eye, generally referred to as mucus, should be slight and transparent, but if it becomes a heavier emission and yellow in colour then this points to excessive intake of dairy products. If a woman has this discoloration and extra discharge in her eyes, then she must expect to have the same density of emission from her vagina.

Even the shape of the nose will give an indication of the Yin and Yang influences. A long thin nose with small nostrils is Yin and caused simply by too much Yin food such as ice cream, imitation fruit drinks, and too many drugs and medicants. A fat bulbous nose shows that the person has an enlarged heart, and if it is also red in colour, then the blood capillaries are under pressure and this could lead to heart trouble or heart disease. A cleft or indentation in the middle of the nose denotes that the two chambers of the heart are not the same size or that they are not working in harmony with one another, and so there is irregular beating which is generally called heart murmur.

What about the mouth? If it is large then this indicates that there is a degeneration in the digestive system and also in the sexual organs. Thin lips or lips of different thickness show that the person is Yin. If the bottom lip is bigger than the top lip then the intestines are in trouble — a very common problem in the West. But if the top lip is swollen then this shows that the stomach is weak. If cuts or cracks appear on the lips then don't waste time — do something about it as soon as you can, or you are going to have bowel trouble. Also ensure that you change your diet if cysts appear on the lips for it can also indicate that you have a cyst, an ulcer or a tumour in the respective region of your organs, the stomach being represented by the top lip, and the large intestine by the bottom lip.

The teeth should all be straight, uniform in size and of a standard shape. If they slope inwards this is a sign of being too Yang; if they slope outwards and have gaps between them, this indicates someone who likes to be on the go and cannot be expected to stay at home for very long. Bad teeth, tooth decay, weak teeth or pointed teeth are all Yin complaints created by bad blood or bad saliva, and all are due to very bad eating and drinking habits.

These are but a few of the many signs of ill health that can be seen on the body, and all that is necessary for diagnosis is a trained eye to recognize the symptons and the ability to know which organ or part of the body is creating the cause. Then one must know how to eradicate the cause, in order to establish good health on a permanent basis.

Using Touch
Diagnosis by touch is the most important section of all, for 'Feeling the Pulse' (K'anmai) or (Chenmai) is an art that every traditional Chinese doctor learns to do first, for it is only acquired by a very delicate and sensitive touch, and experience can only come over a very long period of time and constant practice. It is said that this art goes back to nearly 3000 BC, and it is just as important today as it ever was for it can indicate immediately any irregularities in the functioning of the twelve organs of the body.

Modern Western doctors lay the tip of one finger on the radial artery and count the rhythmic pulsation of the heartbeats. The Chinese doctor places three fingers on the radial artery and by a light pressure can understand the condition of three of the Yang organs, and by a deeper and firmer pressure can appreciate the health of three of the Yin organs. By feeling the pulses on the other wrist, in a similar way, he can obtain information on the differences affecting another six organs, which are as follows:

Left radial artery	Light pressure	Deep pressure
Index finger	Small Intestine	Heart
Middle finger	Gall Bladder	Liver
Third finger	Urinary Bladder	Kidneys

Right radial artery	Light pressure	Deep pressure
Index finger	Large Intestine	Lungs
Middle finger	Stomach	Spleen
Third finger	Triple Heater	Heart Controller

By feeling the pulses, it is possible to understand the levels of internal energy (Ch'i), and there is a vast range of different fluctuations that pass along the channels or meridians connected with the above-mentioned organs. The traditional doctor will then take the necessary steps to sedate or tonify the organs involved.

In addition to the twelve pulses mentioned, there are many other points on the body where the pulse can be taken, such as the arms, neck, head and legs, where the arteries rise fairly close to the surface of the skin.

Touch is also used to feel the strength or weakness, heat or coldness, tension or softness in various parts of the body, and to feel the extent of any lumps or bumps on the surface of the skin or internally, as well as gently feeling the severity of any fractures that have been incurred. So diagnosis through the medium of touch, which is a vast field, is extremely necessary for the full understanding of the human body. Thousands of years of practical experience within China have proved its worth over and over again, and its accuracy amazes Western practitioners.

Using the Ears

The next sense to be used in diagnosis is hearing, or the use of the ears, which can be used to detect alterations in the tones of the voice, the pitch of the voice and whether it is high or low, and whether the tone is smooth or rough. It can detect whether air is entering the lungs smoothly, or whether it has an uneven journey.

The ears can also listen to various internal activities of the body which may be in the form of creaks, clicks or rumblings in the bladder and bowel systems.

Using the Nose
Finally, the nose can be used to help or to confirm diagnosis, for the smell emanating from a person's body through the mouth or armpits, or through the discharge of urine or motions, can indicate the part of the anatomy that is causing the trouble, and will help in the classification of the illness as well.

The 'Eight Classifications'
In addition to these methods of examination, traditional doctors were taught, and are still trained in, the 'Eight Classifications' (Pan Fen Lei), which are also closely related to the Yin and Yang:

1. Yin	2. Yang
3. Internal	4. External
5. Cold	6. Hot
7. Reduced function	8. Increased activity

By fully understanding the meaning and the depth of each, in conjunction with all the five methods of examination and diagnosis, Chinese traditional doctors were able to amalgamate them all into one definite conclusion. Then, and only then, was the appropriate treatment recommended.

Chapter 5

Ch'ang Ming — Taoist Long Life Therapy

Taoist natural health therapy has been a part of the Chinese normal daily life for thousands of years, basically brought into effect by the wisdom and recommendations of the 'Sons of Reflected Light'. Of course, it went through many changes, some of them detrimental to the general health, but it was the Taoists who through the search for physical alchemy finally brought it back to its original form. Since then it has been handed down through every family in the land, and has become a part of the Chinese way of life. Although today the Chinese in various parts of the world have made slight changes, depending on local habits, the fundamentals remain the same.

Most people in the West never think of their health from one day to another, taking it all for granted, so much so that they tend to abuse it in so many different ways, that sooner or later the body can stand no more, and the system breaks down. Youthful vitality will often hide weaknesses that have developed in the human frame. Likewise, if a young child complains of aches and pains, they are often put down to growing pains, and the symptoms ignored. Then as growing older takes its normal course, degeneration and deterioration take place, and eventually the real weaknesses within the framework of the body make their appearance through various symptoms. Then the physical structure, not having the health or the vitality to fight back, slowly wilts under the strain, and the illness spreads more and more.

If you own a house, and allow the roof, the walls and the foundations to deteriorate due to neglect and carelessness through lack of consideration, then eventually it will all collapse, and all you will have left is a pile of worthless rubble. This is what many people do, in this modern age, to their own bodies, and they then wonder why they suffer from sickness and disease in their later lives. It may seem an unfair thing to say, but nevertheless it is true to say that bad health is entirely the sufferer's own fault, even though it might have been caused over the years by lack of understanding and insufficient knowledge.

The Basic Rules of Healthy Eating

In the Western world there is a saying that 'The proof of the pudding is in the eating', but in China all the proof was obtained many thousands of years ago, and it has been well and truly proven through the daily eating habits of the Chinese. These are based on a few simple rules:

1. Eat only when hungry, and not just out of habit.
2. Eat only natural foods.
3. Chew every mouthful of food really well.
4. Don't overeat at any time.
5. Keep your liquid intake down to the barest minimum.

Regarding the first item, the average Chinese eats two good meals every day, and this is ample for survival, for it enables the body to digest the food intake and to distribute it properly through the system, then have a period of rest before the next meal.

Item number two makes common sense in a country with such vast agricultural resources as China, so eating natural and locally grown food makes sense. So you will readily appreciate why the Chinese eat plenty of grain food, vegetables and, to a smaller degree, home-grown fruit.

The third piece of advice — that you should chew the food thoroughly — may seem strange to those in the West who have a tendency to gobble their food, or who constantly wash it down with liquid. They deny themselves the full benefit of their saliva, and they throw an overload onto their digestive systems.

Overeating is another crime against your system, for not only do you swamp your Yang organs so that they cannot digest the food properly, but you do not give them time to complete their work before the next load of food is dumped into them. So is it any wonder that their energies get depleted over a period of time. So reduce your intake of food that is hard to digest, like the white of boiled eggs or meat which has not been cooked thoroughly. The Chinese always cut up all their food into very small pieces, so that any fat or fatty tissues can easily be broken down in the cooking, so it helps to take the strain off the digestive organs.

The fifth item is also extremely important, for too much fluid

Important sources of these vitamins	A	B	B_1	B_2	B_6	B_{12}	C	D	E	K	Calcium	Iron
Wheat	✓	✓	✓	✓	✓				✓	✓	✓	✓
Millet		✓	✓	✓	✓				✓	✓	✓	✓
Rye		✓	✓	✓	✓				✓	✓	✓	✓
Brown rice		✓	✓	✓	✓				✓	✓	✓	✓
Oats		✓	✓	✓	✓				✓	✓	✓	✓
Corn		✓	✓	✓	✓				✓	✓	✓	✓
Broccoli	✓	✓	✓	✓	✓	✓	✓		✓	✓	✓	✓
Cabbage	✓	✓	✓	✓	✓	✓	✓		✓	✓	✓	✓
Peas	✓	✓			✓		✓		✓		✓	✓
Beans	✓	✓			✓		✓		✓		✓	✓
Watercress	✓	✓	✓	✓	✓		✓		✓	✓	✓	✓
Carrots	✓		✓	✓	✓		✓		✓			✓
Kale	✓	✓			✓		✓		✓			✓
Alfalfa	✓	✓			✓		✓		✓			✓
Turnip greens	✓	✓	✓	✓	✓		✓			✓	✓	✓
Beet greens	✓	✓		✓	✓		✓			✓	✓	✓
Mustard greens	✓	✓			✓		✓			✓	✓	✓
Dandelion greens	✓	✓	✓	✓	✓		✓		✓	✓		✓
Tomatoes	✓											
Soya beans	✓	✓	✓	✓	✓		✓		✓	✓	✓	
Seaweed		✓									✓	✓
Sunflower seeds		✓					✓					
Sesame seeds		✓					✓					
Apricots	✓		✓				✓					
Peaches	✓						✓					
Milk		✓		✓							✓	
Fish		✓			✓	✓		✓			✓	
Chicken		✓		✓								
Liver		✓		✓		✓						
Beef		✓		✓	✓	✓						
Lamb		✓			✓	✓						
Pork		✓			✓	✓						
Margarine	✓						✓	✓				
Butter	✓											

in the body can cause enormous damage and also long-term deterioration, and because it is very Yin it is the basic creator of many illnesses. Incidently, very few of the Chinese drink alcohol, although they do make their own wines, which are mainly made from grains, herbs and fruits. Chinese teas are all herb teas, and are always drunk after a meal, and never with a meal or with milk or sugar, and it is a very ancient rule never to have more than three cups at any time, and you know how tiny our Chinese tea-bowls are.

Ch'ang Ming is based on simple rules. Remember that 10,000 years ago the Chinese knew nothing about vitamins A, B, C and D, as they are classified today, but they knew that it was necessary to know the fundamental biological foundations of every food that was grown, including the plant, roots, stalks, leaves, fruits and seeds, as well as all living matter, and to understand what long-term effects each one had upon the human body. So the Taoists experimented upon themselves in their search for physical and spiritual alchemy, and this went on for thousands of years, and many died for the good of the cause. Eventually all practitioners had a very deep understanding of the laws and principles of the universe, and through it the Taoists became very competent dietitians and herbalists.

Chan Kam Lee, in all his wisdom, transferred the basic Taoist recommendations and matched them against the Westernized ways of eating and drinking, nearly sixty years ago, and by balancing the principles of Yin and Yang in line with the food consumed, and then comparing it with the fundamental laws laid down by the Taoists he came up with the chart shown on page 42.

Now compare those items which contain the most vitamins, and have the greatest all-round value that can be offered to the human body, then carefully make a comparison with the Taoist recommendations for sensible eating and drinking habits, which were formulated thousands of years before Christ was born, and you will be amazed just how beneficial these recommendations are to the human body, and all created through the simple understanding of the principles of the Yin and Yang. Now spend a few minutes comparing them

The Taoist Ch'ang Ming Health Diet Recommendations
The following foods can be eaten:

1. You can eat all natural wholegrain foods which have been

organically grown and which have not been refined, including brown rice, wheat, buckwheat, barley, millet, rye, corn, or anything that is made from them such as bread, cakes, puddings, biscuits or breakfast foods.

2. Seaweed.
3. All locally grown vegetables, which are in season, especially root vegetables, peas and beans, but none of those which are mentioned in No. 10 of the foods that are not to be eaten.
4. Bean shoots from soya beans and mung beans.
5. Locally grown nuts (but not salted nuts), preferably roasted.
6. Only locally grown fruit, in season.
7. Low-fat natural yogurt.
8. Honey — but very sparingly.
9. Cottage cheese or vegetarian cheese.
10. Herb teas or China teas.
11. Vegetable margarine, and oils such as sesame or sunflower.
12. Eggs, but only scrambled or in omelettes; better still, the yolk only.
13. Use natural sea salt, or sesame seed salt, or soya sauce.
14. All dried fruit such as cherries, raisins, currants, etc.
15. Grain milk or rice milk — but if necessary, skimmed milk or powdered skimmed milk.
16. Make your own fruit drinks, but only from locally grown fruit, and stay away from commercial and fizzy drinks.
17. Use wild vegetables and herbs whenever you can.
18. Should you wish to do so, you may eat non-fat white fish, birds, poultry and seafoods.

These foods are not to be eaten:

1. Refined or processed foods. If any colourings, preservatives, flavourings, fruit acids or other chemicals are added to the food, don't touch it.
2. Processed grain foods, especially white bread or anything that is made from white flour.
3. Deep fried food.
4. Coffee, alcohol, tobacco, chocolate and other sweets.
5. Spices, rock salt, mustard, pepper, vinegar, pickles or curry.
6. Red meats such as pork, beef, mutton or lamb.
7. Salmon, tuna, mackerel, shark, swordfish or whale.
8. Sugar.
9. Ice cream, artificial jellies, synthetic fruit juices.

10. Potatoes, tomatoes, aubergines, rhubarb and spinach.
11. Concentrated meat extracts, soups or gravies.
12. Cheese, milk, butter; boiled or fried eggs.
13. Lard or dripping that comes from animal fats.
14. Any bird or fish that has a lot of fat tissue.

Processed Foods

Stay away from all foods that contain chemicals and additives, such as artificial colourings, flavourings, preservatives, etc., none of which will do the body any good. In fact, they tend to make the food too Yin or too Yang, and as such, should be avoided at all costs.

Fruit

Even though apples are Yang, fruit generally is Yin and should therefore be eaten in very small quantities. Especially be extremely wary of all tropical fruit such as oranges, figs, pineapples, avocados, papayas, mangoes and bananas, for they are very Yin indeed. So, contrary to popular Western belief, it is inadvisable to give a sick person fruit as a present, as it is likely not only to upset the complaint, but to retard the activeness of the body mechanism, and therefore make the body take longer to heal itself.

Vegetables

Use only those that are grown locally and that happen to be in season at the time, preferably those grown organically. Pulses such as peas, beans and lentils are especially good, since they are rich in protein, iron and many vitamins. Did you know that watercress, green peppers, cauliflowers, cabbage and brussels sprouts all contain more vitamin C than oranges? Carrots, watercress and dried apricots contain the highest quantities of vitamin A, whilst dry lentils, dried apricots, dried figs, almonds, oatmeal, wholemeal and chicken all give quite good amounts of iron, which is so necessary for the red pigment of the blood.

Herbs

Though herbs tend not to be used to the same extent that they used to be, they are still reasonably cheap, and very beneficial to the general health of the body. There are so many that it would take many books to cover all the herbs of the world, but some of the more common ones like sage, burdock, thyme, parsley, watercress, dandelion, basil and bay leaf can be added to food and soups, for they all have excellent qualities, and each will add its own flavour to the food. They can all be taken as an infusion, and they do make a very pleasant drink, once you get used to their individual flavours.

Rice
White rice has been polished, and in some cases may have also been bleached. So it is much better to buy brown rice, which, while taking a little longer to cook, will retain the goodness normally lost during processing. Short grain brown is the best.

Grains
All grains and cereals contain high levels of energy and give good quantities of protein, calcium and iron, and they may be consumed in a wide variety of different ways. Not only can they be used as food, but they can also make excellent milk, as well as other beverages. By browning any grain, including brown rice, in a frying pan, then adding water and boiling the mixture, a very pleasant drink can be made. Add honey or soya sauce to suit your own taste.

Fish
Once a week is more than enough to eat fish or any other seafood. This is because all fish and seafood is very Yin, so not only should it be eaten in small quantities, but also not too often.

Meats
No meat is really necessary for the human body as all the nourishment that is required can be obtained from grains and vegetables. In addition to this, meat and animal fats are very difficult for the stomach to digest, and therefore tend to create an overload on the whole digestive system. They create toxin, which is bad for the circulation and nervous system.

Salt
Ordinary salt contains very little goodness, as most of it evaporated with the water millions of years ago, but sea salt does retain various minerals as well as traces of iodine, all of which are utilized by the human body. However, anyone over 50 years of age should reduce salt intake, for high salt intake is known to be associated with high blood-pressure. One of the best condiments is sesame salt, a mixture of nine parts ground sesame seeds with one part sea salt. It is available in most health food shops, or you can easily make it yourself.

Potatoes, Tomatoes and Aubergines
These are related to Belladonna (Deadly Nightshade), and they share some of its deadly properties deriving from the alkaloid of solanine poison, and so are best left out of your diet.

Rhubarb and Spinach
Both contain soluble oxalic poison, so again it is recommended that these should be left out of the diet.

Chocolate, Coffee and Tea
Few people are aware of the harmful effects of these drinks, for they contain caffeine, tannin and other harmful ingredients, and because they tend to act as stimulants they can throw a strain upon the heart. Chocolate on the other hand, is one of the causes of acne in children, and in addition to that, it also tends to reduce the amount of calcium entering into the body, so thereby creating weaknesses in the teeth, nails and bones.

Ch'ang Ming can help everyone to retain constant good health and it will help the very thin person to put on weight, and it will assist those suffering from obesity to slim down to a more natural body weight, thereby conforming to the natural laws of the universe. It will overcome all diseases, and will heal all sickness, by the very simple process of making the body and all its organs strong and truly efficient, so that it eventually cures itself.

How can Ch'ang Ming help you to maintain good health, and also ensure that the sick and suffering can regain it? Firstly, it ensures that the organs of the body are able to work one hundred per cent efficiently, and to do this it is necessary to get rid of the surplus fat, excess water, toxins and acidity that have been allowed to accumulate within the body. Ch'ang Ming will do this quite easily, providing you are willing to change your eating and drinking habits. It means, of course, that you may have to give up certain things that you enjoy, and sometimes learn to eat and drink other things that you have previously disliked.

We have also to ensure that the digestive system is working efficiently, so that the food consumed is digested well and dispersed as quickly as possible. The bowels must also be emptied daily, so that any poisonous matter is not retained within the body for too long a period, and we must endeavour to help this disposal and removal.

The blood plays an important part in the body, so it is essential that it is of the right composition, and it does its job within the circulatory system. Of course, there should be no blockages or restrictions in the circulation, and if there are, then these will have to be cleared away, so that the various glands, veins and junctions in the system do their job really well and free from hindrance and obstruction, so that nothing will impede their action. In cases of arthritis we must also wash the alkaline away from the affected joints, so that Ch'ang Ming can truly help the body to speed up the process of making new bone and new skin tissue.

A further aspect of Wu Hsing (the Five Elements) is found in the five stages that all patients must go through if they are truly dedicated to achieving complete recovery from illness, and aim for constant good health for the rest of their lifespan here on this earth. Even those who are not quite so dedicated as others can go through at least four stages of recovery as follows:

1. Purification: This cleanses the internal and external parts of the body by getting rid of acidity, toxins and all the poisonous matter, and this includes the effects of drugs that may still be retained within the system.
2. Activation: This stage is the start of healing and the beginning of obtaining good health, through the simple expedient of awakening all parts of the body and making them commence to do their work with maximum efficiency. This is between one month and six weeks after starting on a Ch'ang Ming diet.
3. Cultivation: With all the internal organs now working correctly the body now goes ahead to create new skin tissue, throughout all the organs, as well as within the flesh and muscles. This takes about three years.
4. Creation: This carries on the work from Stage 3 and starts to renew all the nails, teeth and bones. This stage can take up to ten years.
5. Occlusion: This stage concentrates on the retention of permanent good health, and on increasing one's lifespan. (See Chapter 13 on this subject.)

So the whole essence of constant good health is completely dependent upon eating the right foods, as our ancestors did before us, more than ten thousand years ago, and ensuring that the foods that we consume in our daily lives are completely natural.

But what are natural foods? Mention natural foods to the average man in the street and he will think that you are a faddist or a quack, but he has overlooked the fact that natural food has always been the lifeline of humanity, and that it was the sort of food consumed by his own grandparents and their grandparents before them. Natural food is organically grown, without the use of fertilizers or pesticides, and it is completely unprocessed, and thereby retains its natural nutritional constituents.

It has only been in the last few decades that chemicals have become more widely used: pesticides, fertilizers, bleaches, additives, colourings, preservatives, flavourings, in highly refined foods, or in packaged goods. Even many imported fruits are automatically sprayed with preservatives before they are exported, and if you don't wash that fruit in hot water before you eat it, then you get more chemicals in your system.

So Ch'ang Ming will not only cure sickness of all kinds, but will also ensure that you never become ill again, by the simple process of making the body do its work properly, and making it strong again, so that it can cure itself and fight off any infection. After all, the Supreme Spirit (Yuhuang Tati) made the human body in such a way that it should be able to fulfil this function continuously, easily and automatically. If it fails to do so, then you have to give it a helping hand to enable it to do the job that it was made to do in the first place, and to do it really efficiently.

That is Ch'ang Ming (Taoist natural health and long life therapy) in a nutshell, but don't bother with it unless you are fully prepared to dedicate yourself to the task, and you truly and sincerely want to be cured, once and for all. It may only take a few weeks to achieve your target or it may take a few years, depending on the current state of your health. Whatever the case, the effort must be yours. It all depends entirely upon you. Good health will only be achieved through dedication and the sincere desire to get well. It is your natural heritage, but you must work conscientiously to reclaim it.

Chapter 6

Ts'ao Yao — Chinese Herbal Therapy

Throughout history, man has appreciated the importance of the vegetable kingdom in his life. It has provided him with food, clothing and numerous other products. In addition it has played an important part in the international economy. Thousands of years ago, medicinal herbs were being transported across China and India, and onwards to the Middle East and the Mediterranean countries. The Chinese fostered a very lucrative export business, in both herbs and other merchandise, through the many traders who dared to risk their lives on the long trek over desert plains, high mountains, dense jungle and along very poor tracks. The Chinese, then, have long been associated with herbal medicine and its spread throughout the world.

Through the infinite wisdom and teachings of the 'Sons of Reflected Light', the Chinese were given a really wonderful start and a unique foundation to their knowledge by being taught how to explore the great depths of herbal therapy, making possible the development of its vast potential in preventative and curative medicine. It was Shen Nung, however, later more popularly known as Huang Ti (The Yellow Emperor), the second emperor of China, who is said to have been the first to tabulate the useful and harmful properties of hundreds of herbs.

Shen Nung lived in about 3000 BC, and is said to have been influenced by the element of Fire (Huo). He has always been credited with the invention of the plough, the construction of the first wheeled cart, formulating various systems of irrigation, and furthering the understanding of husbandry, in addition to his highly valuable work with herbs.

After his death, Shen Nung was chosen to be one of the gods of the apothecaries of China, and was given the title of 'The Divine Husbandman'. His classic of internal medicine, the *Nei Ching*, is well known all over the world, and is still used by traditional doctors and modern physicians as a book of reference, although it has since been divided into two main sections, the Su Wen and the Ling Shu. The complete work covers twenty-four books and a total of eighty-one chapters.

Since the reign of the Yellow Emperor the tremendous work of listing over 30,000 herbs used in traditional medicine has steadily grown, but they are also listed under the properties of their roots and tubers, leaves and stalks, fruit and seeds, as well as the vast range of prescriptions that are available.

One of the most important works on this subject was written by Li Shih Chen, with over 12,000 herbs and herbal prescriptions. It was first published in China in the sixteenth century. Not only was he a traditional doctor, but he was also a qualified herbalist and pharmacologist, and his writings, which were called the *Compendium of Remedies (Pen Ts'ao Kang Mu)*, were the result of nearly thirty years of experience and practical work.

Even today in this modern world, the Western professions are quite surprised at the extraordinary number of herbal combinations that not only exist in writing in China, but are still used extensively by traditional doctors for the prevention and cure of so many illnesses. What many people do not fully appreciate is that all the herbs are also affected by the influence of Yin and Yang, for they can be used either internally or externally, and sometimes simultaneously. The results obtained over thousands of years have been well and truly proven, but naturally everything depends on their proper use, as well as a full understanding of their sphere of influence, their effects and whether they are of long or short duration, and also the length of time for which they can be administered.

For instance, when being used internally, they can be taken in the form of pills, powders, hot or cold drinks or soups, dependent on the particular illness being treated. For other complaints they may have to be administered before or after a meal, and sometimes in the very early morning before any food passes the lips, or it may be necessary to take them in the late evening after the last meal has been digested. Then it is necessary to consider whether an immediate effect is required, or whether it is necessary to have a slow progression over a much longer period.

The external working potential of all herbs has to be considered on the same basis. One must ask whether it is necessary to have a hot or cold application, or both, each following the other. If the latter, one must know what time-limits have to be adhered to, for long or short periods have to be considered, as each herb has its different characteristics. Some can penetrate quite deeply below the surface of the skin, while others only exert their influence to a point just below the surface. Then there is a further consideration to be made, namely, whether the application should cover as big an area as possible, or whether it will suffice to concentrate the herb's potential on a very small spot.

Whilst the internal is Yin and the external is Yang, everything listed above has its dual role to be considered, and because of this it will have a dual effect in its work, and in the results that are obtained in its application. That is why it is important that people living in the colder climates (Yin) should concentrate on eating more Yang foods, and those living in the tropical areas (Yang) should endeavour to consume more Yin foods.

The ancient and traditional herbal textbooks generally classify herbs into five categories, in conformity with the 'Five Elements' (Wu Hsing) as follows:

1. Those that are nutritious and can be eaten daily with a normal Ch'ang Ming diet.
2. Non-poisonous herbs that can be used in medicines.
3. Poisonous herbs that must only be used in very small quantities.
4. Those herbs that can only be used for a short period of time.
5. Those herbs that can safely be used over long periods of time

The majority of herbs that are grown in the West are also known and found in China. This is due to its great geographical diversity, which includes mountains in the north, tropical regions in the south, deserts in the west and a long coastline in the east. On the other hand, there are many herbs which are grown in China and yet which are unknown in the West.

Let us now list some of the herbs that can be used to assist nature in the task of obtaining the right balance within the human body, so that the cause of an illness can be eradicated.

Pearl barley (Imi) — *Coix lachryma jobi L.*
This is quite pleasant to the taste, and it has a very cooling influence on the system. It will help to strengthen the spleen, combat diarrhoea and lung abscesses, and is excellent for pneumonia and appendicitis; and because it has a tendency to convert moisture within the human body it is of great benefit to all those who have difficulty in passing urine.

Mugwort (Ai yen) — *Artemisia vulgaris*
One of the very ancient herbs of China, it is also very common in other parts of the world, where it abounds in the countryside. The leaves and the roots can be used internally where it will act as a stimulant, and it can also be used externally on the skin, in the form of a poultice on aching joints and for muscular pains. It can also be taken as an infusion, but only in small quantities, and it will stop internal bleeding, stimulate the appetite, help to regulate menstruation, restore energy levels, dispel wind and abdominal cramps, and will also clear up a variety of skin complaints.

Celery (Han ch'in) — *Apium graveolens*
This is the wild variety, which, taken as a drink, is extremely useful in calming hysteria. Its soothing properties will also help to promote relaxation, physically and mentally, and a good night's sleep. Because it contains two different oils, one heavy and one light, it has a tendency to neutralize uric acid, and therefore it is excellent in the fight against rheumatism, arthritis and gout. It has a very pleasant smell, and although the flower itself might seem a little flat to look at, it is very warming to the physical system.

Pride of China (K'u lien) — *Melia azadirachta*
This tree is native to China, but due to the export of its nuts, it can now be found growing in India, Spain and southern France. The nuts are very hard indeed, so have been used in the making of rosaries for many centuries. They are poisonous and are never eaten. It is the bark of the tree, however, that has the unique properties that make it an excellent medicant. When taken as a drink, it acts as a dynamic purgative, so much so that it can rid the system of worms more quickly than most other remedies.

Plantain (Ch'e ch'ien) — *Plantago major L.*
I wonder how many gardeners in the world curse this very common weed, which is just as common in China as anywhere else, and multiplies just as quickly. It is used, and very successfully, for all external inflammations, such as nettle stings, insect stings and bites, and morbid skin complaints caused by heat, friction or pain, as well as for cuts, grazes and external haemorrhages. Internally it is used to combat consumption, dysentery and bleeding of the stomach and lungs.

Bengal madder (Hsi ts'ao) — *Rubia cordifolia L.*
A creeping perennial plant which grows mainly in China and India, and which loves the dampness that is found in thick undergrowth and in the jungles. Only the roots are used medicinally, for they contain rubianic acid, which is soluble in hot water. Whilst it is quite bitter to the taste it does have excellent cooling properties. Because of this, it has been found to be extremely useful in the fight against rheumatoid arthritis, abdominal pains and jaundice, because it quickly reduces internal inflammation.

Sage (Sheng jen) — *Salvia officinalis*
So many Westerners have forgotten the benefits of this herb and only consider it worthy to stuff the chicken or turkey with at Christmas time. Its many properties warrant it a much worthier place in the household than that, for the herb is extremely beneficial to the system as a whole. It soothes the stomach, tonifies the intestines, aids weak digestion, helps those who have lost their appetite, stops internal bleeding, and is very good for kidney and liver troubles, as well as colds. It will relieve the sweating of those suffering from influenza and tuberculosis. External cuts, grazes, bruises and any knocks or sprains can be soothed by bathing the area of the skin with an infusion of this herb. Use it more in your daily life and you will find it truly worth your while. Get into the habit of always keeping some in the kitchen or in your first-aid box.

Chinese rose (Yeuh chi hua) — *Rosa Chinensis Jacq.*
This grows mainly in southern China, and it normally blooms all the year round, which is wonderful from a medicinal point of view, as it is the flowers that are mainly used. It helps irregular menstruation and menstrual pains, and it will greatly help the smooth flowing of the blood in the circulation system of the body. It is also excellent for serious injuries to the body, especially the back of the trunk.

Dandelion (P'u kung ying) — *Taraxacum officinale*
In its wild state this herb seems to grow everywhere in the world, yet there are only two countries that seem to cultivate it properly for its true worth, and they are China and France, where its virtues are fully put to proper use, in food as well as medication. It has a high vitamin A and vitamin C content, and it contains more iron than spinach, as well as many other valuable constituents. In China

we use the whole plant for medicinal purposes. As a tea it has a rather bitter taste, but the root, when roasted and ground, makes an excellent coffee which can be drunk by children, the elderly and the sick at any time. Taken at night-time just before retiring, it will soothe the system, and thereby encourage the body to have a deep and restful sleep.

It also has a wonderful effect on the kidneys, bladder and stomach, and it will quickly clear the skin of boils and abscesses. It will help nursing mothers to generate more milk for their babies. Because it has a rather cooling effect on the body, it is used quite extensively to dispel fevers and high temperatures.

Chinese yam (Shan yao) — *Dioscorea batatas decne*
Only the long angular stem tubers are used in Chinese herbal therapy, and when they are used as an infusion they give the tea a rather sweetish taste. The tubers contain many soluble fats, starch, glutamine, and quite a number of amino acids. It nourishes the lungs, kidneys, stomach, spleen and pancreas, and therefore it is used to combat asthma, bronchitis and emphysema. In addition anyone suffering from chronic enteritis or dysentery will find this herb of enormous benefit, as will those who suffer from leucorrhoea and those who tend to be neurotic.

Tarragon (Ch'ing hao) — *Artemisia dracunculus*
Sometimes this is known as the 'little dragon' and it has extensive usage in China, not only as a herb for medicants, but also added to vinegar to give it flavour. It is also found in tartare sauce, French dressing and mayonnaise. Medicinally this herb is excellent for the heart, brain and liver, due mainly to the volatile oil it contains.

Knotgrass (Pien hsu) — *Polygonum aviculaire L.*
Every part of this annual weed is used quite extensively in Chinese medicinal practice. On its own it can be made into a tea by using one ounce to one pint of boiling water, then allowing it to cool before drinking. It quickly clears fevers, and it also has a tendency to dry up excess moisture in the body. It eradicates urinary stones and their formation, and is really excellent for women who have an excess discharge of mucus from the vagina.

It is also used to combat inflammation of the pelvis or the kidney, which medically is commonly known as pyelitis, and in the case of diuresis it will help enormously to regulate the flow of the urine.

Vervain (Ma pien ts'ao) — *Verbena officinalis*
This wild perennial herb is sometimes also mistaken for lemon verbena, but the latter does have a very distinctive lemon smell and flavour, and it is not as hardy as the wild vervain. Vervain was used extensively in England during the plague, and has also been included in various love potions up to the eighteenth century.

Slightly bitter to the palate it has been found to strengthen the nerves, and acts as a soothant to bronchial congestion. It brings fast relief to the migraine headache, and also those which might be caused by stress, worry, tension and fatigue. It will also combat infections in the urinary tract, with extreme efficiency, and also in the liver, the latter being known as hepatitis. Women who suffer from amenorrhoea, when the menstrual flow ceases, will find this particular herb very beneficial, as will those with inflammation of the breast.

The whole plant is used in Chinese herbalism, and it can be used fresh or as a dried herb, and when used as a tea it can be taken either hot or cold.

Cloves (Ting hsiang) — *Eugenia caryophyllata Thunb.*
Cloves have been used in cakes, puddings and sweets for many centuries, and most people will find them a bit strong and spicy. They contain quite a large amount of essential oil in the form of volatile oil, which is used extensively in Chinese medicine. It is quite a powerful antiseptic, and will greatly assist people who have lazy bowel systems and constant flatulence. It can also be used with great success against pulmonary tuberculosis and bronchitis.

Because it has such a warming effect on the body, it helps to alleviate pain, and those illnesses caused through internal coldness.

Burra Gookero (Chi li) — *Tribulis terrestris L.*
Only the fruits are used in Chinese herbalism. When ripened they turn to a deep brown. These fruits contain two separate cells which give birth to four long and narrow seeds, which can be made into a bitter-tasting infusion. Because the bitterness is so strong, the tea is normally made up of only one part of the seeds to twenty parts of water.

It is mainly used for complaints of men, such as incontinence, nocturnal emissions, gonorrhoea and impotence. It does have some very useful properties which neutralize acidity within the liver and help to dispel wind. It severely restricts excess moisture in the body, and therefore it has been found to be excellent for those who suffer from various lung complaints, and which generally show up as nose and throat ailments.

Camphor (Chang) — *Cinnamonum camphora (T. Nees and Eberm)*
The white crystalline oil which comes from this evergreen tree has been very highly valued by the Chinese for thousands of years, not only for medicinal purposes but also for embalming, including the oil in the manufacture of soap to give it an aromatic scent, and for making Chinese inks and artists colourings.

The whole plant can be used medicinally, including the bark and the roots, but it must be given only in small doses as it can prove to be poisonous in large amounts. It has 'heat' properties, which help to stimulate the blood and the circulation of Ch'i energy, and because of this, it is excellent for complaints of the stomach, abdominal pains and the bowel system. It alleviates all kinds of pain, such as toothache, injuries that may have been incurred in accidents, sprains and other muscular stresses, and it has also been found invaluable in the fight against rheumatism, osteoarthritis, cholera and beri-beri. (I have ample personal evidence for this. I was a prisoner of war of the Japanese, in the jungles of Burma for three years, and whilst many other prisoners died from malnutrition, malaria, cholera and beri-beri, I never got a single attack of illness, because I was able to find many herbs, and also managed to scrounge, from time to time, some camphor from the local men and women who had been conscripted into the working parties. When I finally managed to escape, I was nearly down to six stone in weight, but I had retained my good health.)

As you have read, camphor when taken in large doses can be poisonous to the system, and this also applies to many other plants. You are no doubt aware of the fact that there are many other poisonous plants, which should never be eaten or drunk in teas under normal circumstances, but which when taken in small doses, under strict medical control, can be used to combat various forms of sickness and disease. Here are a few of these poisonous plants that are used in China to combat the weaknesses that have developed within the human body:

Potato (Maling shu) — *Solanum tuberosum*
The potato is very commonly cultivated and eaten in the Western world and in very large quantities, but even so, it is not very widely known that this plant has a poisonous constituent which is known as glyco-alkaloid, which has caused many severe illnesses, and in

some cases death, in animals and humans.

However, the potato, when it is grated and the juice squeezed out, or cut into small pieces, boiled in a small quantity of water, then filtered through a very fine mesh cloth, gives a creamy-coloured water which has beneficial properties. When drunk in small quantities before a meal it helps to combat stomach acidity, and uric acid for those who suffer from arthritis, and also gastric ulcers. If you find it unpalatable in its raw state, a little drop of soya sauce or honey may be added to it, or the potato juice can be added to soup. But only drink this for a period of four to six weeks.

Black nightshade (Lung kuei) — *Solanum nigrum*

This is the same family as the potato, and therefore it has the same poisonous constituent, namely glyco-alkaloid, and because it grows wild, and has very inviting black berries, it can be extremely dangerous to children. Tests in China have proved that it can be fatal even to livestock.

However, whilst the whole plant is used medicinally after it has been boiled, it is the juice that is used in minute dosages in our ancient herbalism. It is mainly used to clear various types of fevers, to assist the body to pass urine, and to eliminate toxic levels in the system. Because of this, it is an internal aid against external symptoms which show themselves in the form of skin ulcers, rashes, boils etc. It is also a very powerful weapon in the fight against leucorrhoea.

Tomato (Fanch'ie) — *Lycopersicum esculentum*

This is another poisonous plant which contains solanine alkaloids, and is also a distant cousin of the potato, the deadly nightshade and the black nightshade. In the West, of course, it is very widely cultivated for its fruits.

It has been said and written that tomatoes cause or encourage the growth of cancer, but there is as yet no definite proof of this assumption, although it has been proved in tests on animals that they can cause gastro-enteritis, apathy, nervous complaints, and other illnesses of various kinds.

In our ancient Chinese medicine, the whole plant is used, but any dosages that are given are always in very small quantities. It is used to fight against excess toxification in the stomach, enlarged thyroid glands, feverish attacks of all kinds, and also leucorrhoea.

Caper spurge (Hsu sui tze) — *Euphorbia lathyrus*
Every part of this herbaceous biennial plant is poisonous — roots, stem, leaves and seeds. The poisoning is extremely severe with drastic effects, including serious blistering of the intestinal tract, inflammation and irritation of the skin, and even death. This herb is no longer used in Europe, but in China it is still being used as a purgative, and when it is mixed with other herbs, it has proved to be very effective for internal and external swellings of the body, as well as ulcers and dropsy. However, only the oil from the plant is used for medicinal purposes, and then only in minute quantities.

Rhubarb (Ta huang) — *Rheum officinale*
This perennial plant is also well known in the West, but it is less well known that it contains soluble oxalate poison which can cause vomiting and diarrhoea, and severe blood-clotting. Even fatality is not unknown, especially after the leaves have been consumed. However, when used with extreme care by qualified herbalists it can be used in the treatment of ulcers, dropsy, constipation, inflammation of the throat, and even heart disease.

Opium poppy (P'ai hua ying su) — *Papaver somniferum*
This annual plant, whilst being cultivated in many parts of the world, does have a white variety which grows wild in many places, including eastern England. Most people are under the impression that it is the seed of this plant that supplies opium, but in actual fact it is only the husk of the seed that contains it. However, the rest of the plant does contain alkaloid poisons which can slowly destroy the body by restricting the circulation of the blood, cause irregular respiration, create deep contraction of the pupils, very heavy sleep from which it is difficult to awake, and a very deep thirst.

Yet on the other hand the alkaloid of this plant supplies both morphine and codeine, both of which are now widely used and known in modern medicine, and which can be used on their own or in conjunction with other medicants.

Chapter 7

Wen Chiech'u — Thermogenesis

The *Nei Ching* says that 'all generations should hold in awe the beneficial applications of heat treatment which can help the exterior and also aid the interior of the body,' and how true these words are, even in this day and age, when many applications of herbal and non-herbal heat treatments are being used to combat both serious and minor illnesses.

Many different kinds of heat treatments have, through the centuries, been used by the nations of the world, but they were mainly in the form of hot or cold water or applied with hot sticks or pokers. China, however, went into this field to a far deeper extent than most countries, and this was due entirely to the foundations which were laid down by the 'Sons of Reflected Light'. So it is today that there is a vast field of hot and cold therapy available to all traditional Chinese doctors whether they practise ancient or modern medicine, to expedite relief or to speed up the processes of healing.

Recognition of the healing properties of heat goes back many thousands of years, as we already know, so a very firm basis had already been formulated before the *Nei Ching* had been written. It was an integral part of our ancient Chinese philosophy that if Yin was trapped inside, then it could only be released by Yang on the outside, and when Yin endeavours to work its way outward, then the balance can only be controlled by the Yang being made to work its way inward.

In every aspect of Chinese healing the aim is to achieve the harmonious balance of Yin and Yang within the human body, and should any man or woman, accumulate too much of one or not enough of the other, then the Chinese doctor will endeavour to attain the ultimate balance between the two extremes so that good health can be restored once more. What one man can do through bad eating and drinking habits, other men can undo by ancient methods and deep understanding.

On these principles Chinese Wen Chiech'u (heat treatment) is based, and there are many different ways that it can be applied, so all sick and suffering can receive its benefits.

Moxabustion (Aichiu)

No one really knows how long this form of heat treatment has been used in China, but certainly it goes back a long time before the primitive period of oriental history, which was thousands of years before Stone Age man became known in Europe. So it is very ancient indeed. It is known that this form of treatment was used by the people of the northern area of China more than by the people living in the southern regions. This was due, no doubt, to the colder atmosphere, bitter winds, ice and snow, which in turn created the wet and damp weather and caused many internal health problems unknown in the hot tropical southern districts. It is a perfect example and indication of the many ways in which Yin illnesses can be balanced and harmonized by correct Yang influence.

Ai is the Chinese word for the mugwort plant (*Artemisia vulgaris*), and in the West it is also known as St John's plant, and felon herb, whereas in China, depending on the particular area, it may be called mountain mugwort (chan ai) or fine mugwort (sheng ai). *Chiu* is the Chinese word meaning cauterization, which our dictionary specifies as a process of searing or burning the skin tissue through the use of a hot iron, so *Aichiu* is technically a Chinese heat treatment by burning, and generally referred to in the West as moxabustion.

Whereas acupuncture (Hsia Chen Pien) which is a cold process (Yin) and therefore mainly used to combat illnesses caused by an excess of Yang, Aichiu on the other hand, being a hot remedy (Yang) is used to reduce the Yin excesses. Although Aichiu is a complete art within itself, and has a very long tradition in its own right, it has been associated with acupuncture for many centuries. Whilst both can be used separately, they are often used together, as well as being used separately but applied one after the other.

Aichiu is made from the pulverized leaves of the mugwort plant, but only the down (the soft, hairy growth which is on the underside of the leaves) is actually used, and this is separated by heating and then rubbing the leaves between both hands until only the thin fibres, which look like cotton threads, remain. At one time the down was then placed on the skin of the patient, lit, and then allowed to smoulder, thereby creating sufficient heat for the treatment.

Unfortunately, this form of treatment left the patient with some

very ugly scars, and even to this day many of the older generation
bear witness to this mode of heat therapy. However, in this modern
era, there is no longer the danger of burning or singeing of the
skin tissue. This is because a new technique is used: the herb is
wrapped in special paper or compressed tightly into very small
tubes, and then ignited to create the warmth required; then, instead
of placing it in direct contact with the skin, it is held just above
a specific point on the line of the meridian (Ching Hsien Tu) that
is to be treated.

While the use of Aichiu is extremely powerful and very effective,
there are certain points on the body on which this form of treatment
should never be used. Nor should other form of heat therapy be
used on these points. All those who wish to practise any form of
heat treatment should carefully memorize these forbidden points.

Modern doctors are apt to consider that the sole object of Aichiu
heat therapy is to stimulate the exterior of the skin. This attitude
shows the limitations that encompass the Western medical
profession, and invariably they retard their advancement into a
world where natural progress comes by following the Way (Tao),
and the ordained way of all things that live and grow within the
universe.

In Aichiu, the heat acts as a stimulant to the skin, and assists
the curative properties of the herb in their deep penetration.
Through the heat that is generated, the internal energy (Sheng Chi)
is activated into a flowing movement down the lines of the meridians
(Ching Hsein Tu), and in turn passes on to the various connecting
organs to which they are associated. In addition to these benefits,
the heat also influences the blood and the tissue in the immediate
vicinity where the application is being applied, so that the
circulation is strongly increased, and the natural oils of the body
are drawn to that particular area.

So the mugwort herb has a very diverse beneficial influence on
the human body, and its versatility is its main property. However,
there is one inconvenience with this treatment, owing to the burning
and smouldering of the Ai herb, for the aromatic smoke can be
a little overpowering for those who are not used to it. It is therefore
essential that the ventilation of the room is good, and yet not subject
to drafts.

The down of the Ai is normally moulded into bean-sized cones,
small balls, short thin tubes or sticks, and their uses depend upon
the condition of the patient. If only a warming effect is required,
then the sticks are invariably used, but if the complaint is more

serious and a greater heat is required, then the Ai, in the form of a cone or ball, will be placed directly onto the skin, and it is quite possible that three to five of these cones or balls might be burned during a treatment session, which might last up to twenty minutes.

However, if we want to increase the heat potential of the Aichiu, then powdered sea salt (Hai Yen) is placed on the area of the skin where treatment is required, and then the Ai is placed on the top of it, and allowed to smoulder. Great care must be taken, however, for the salt gets very hot, so a strict watch must be kept in case the salt should cause blisters to form.

This same principle is also used when utilizing the benefits of ginger (Chiang), garlic (Ta Suan), cabbage leaves (Paitsai Ye), soya bean cheese (Tatou Kanlao), and many others, when we want the Ai and accompanying herbs to do a specific job, or to cause deeper penetration, or to increase activation of the internal energy (Sheng Chi) of the body, so that a more positive result can be achieved.

Cupping (Pa Hua Kuan)

This is a very simple method of helping to heal arthritis, abdominal pains, paralysis caused by a stroke, abscesses, and other illnesses caused through being out in the cold weather and catching internal chills. However, it should not be used on pregnant women, as it works on the principle of a very strong drawing action, similar to a type of suction, created by a vacuum.

Generally cups or glasses are used, the latter being the most common these days. They consist of two sizes. The larger one is for the very fleshy parts of the body such as the thigh or the abdomen, and for young people. The smaller size will be used on parts of the body which are less fleshy, such as the joints, and for the older generation, or for the very weak person, or for very young children. In the old days, bamboo was used for this purpose, but it was necessary to rub the edges of the wood on a fine stone to give it a smooth surface when making contact. Bamboo has the advantage of holding the heat longer within the vacuum created.

The practitioner soaks in alcohol a ball of cotton wool, a sponge, herbs or just paper. The material is then lit and put inside the receptacle, using a pair of tweezers or forceps. Once the oxygen inside the cup has been absorbed, and a certain degree of heat has been attained, a vacuum is created inside the cup. The flaming material is then withdrawn. Then, providing the edges of the cup or glass are not too hot, so that it will not burn or damage the skin tissue, it can then be placed on the body of the patient, on the spot that has been previously chosen for the treatment.

In the majority of cases, the patient will be made to lie down before the cupping process commences. The length of time the treatment will last is normally in the region of ten to fifteen minutes. This is generally sufficient for the circulation of the body to be induced into the area, and it can be seen very easily as reddish stripes appear faintly on the surface of the skin tissues.

The cup or glass is removed by gently depressing the skin near to the lips of the utensil, allowing air into it, then slowly tipping it to one side. It will then release itself from the tissue quite easily. The next step is to lightly smear the surface of the skin with a little oil (sesame oil is the best) or ointment, which will have a soothing effect.

Blood-Drawing (Hsieh La)

This conforms to the same procedure as the normal cupping treatment, with the exception that the skin is first lightly punctured to allow a very small amount of blood to be discharged. The area is then immediately cupped, and this will draw a considerable amount of blood into the cup. This treatment is only used in extreme cases of strokes, high blood-pressure, stings and snake bites.

Blood-Letting (Ch'ao Hsieh)

Whilst this is not a part of the art of thermogenesis (Wen Chiech'u) it is mentioned here because the technique is very similar to the art of blood-drawing (Hsieh La). Blood-letting is a very simple method which involves pricking the skin with a triangular needle or magnetic disk, just sufficiently to allow a minute amount of blood to pass out. It is executed at specific points of the body to combat certain complaints, such as sunstroke or heatstroke, colic, diarrhoea, vomiting, abscesses, nervous shock, and some bodily injuries. In this art, cupping is unnecessary, because only a very small amount of blood is required to be released.

Hot Baths (Jo Hsi Tsao)

A good hot bath is a wonderful aid in the promotion of good health, for it helps to get rid of toxins in the body, through the pores of skin, and indirectly through the vibrations that are set up in this type of contact heat therapy. Through these contact heat vibrations such organs as the kidneys and the liver receive indirect massage which tones them up, and thereby their work becomes more efficient. Hot baths are very relaxing and a great benefit to a good night's sleep, and they also assist in the promotion of good blood circulation.

Such baths are excellent for those who suffer from rheumatism, cramps, blood stagnation and internal congestions, but anyone with a weak heart should ensure that the water is only warm and *not* hot. You can lie in the bath from fifteen to thirty minutes, but when doing so, ensure that the whole body is immersed, from the tips of the toes to the nape of the neck. Foam headrests are now available from most hardware stores and this will save the back of the head from becoming sore, and bath mats which have suckers underneath are excellent for the older person, who might be a little apprehensive about the possibility of sliding down the bath.

Sea Salt Baths (Haiyan Hsitsao)

Everyone knows the benefit of bathing in the sea for certain ailments, and these results can be obtained just as easily at home by simply adding sea salt to the bath water. This is excellent for those who suffer from glandular disturbances, which will generally show themselves in the form of obesity. These baths will also help to increase blood circulation, and will also help to eliminate thyroid troubles and goitres.

About three or four handfuls of sea salt should be sufficient, and melting the salt in a pan of hot water before having a bath, and tipping it into the bath water, will ensure that you gain the maximum benefit. Don't use any soap or baths salts as this will turn to scum and will float on the top of the water. Lay in this sea salt bath for period of twenty to thirty minutes to really help your complaints.

Epsom Salts Baths (Hsieh Yen Hsi Tsao)

It is possible to purchase commercial Epsom Salts, which is reasonably cheap in price, from most chemist shops and all you need to do is to put two tumblersful in your hot bath water, and then lay in it for a minimum of twenty minutes. At the end of this period scrub the surface of the skin with a good stiff brush, and you will gain the maximum benefit from this insertion. Now run the water out of the bath, then refill it with warm clean water, and thoroughly rinse yourself down, or get under a warm shower. Now dry yourself off and go straight to bed. Rheumatics, arthritics, and those suffering from muscular cramps will gain great benefit from this type of bath.

Ginger Baths (Chiang Hsi Tsao)

Take 1 lb of ginger root powder, and place it in a cotton bag and tie the top with string. Then place the bag into the largest pan that you have, preferably one that will hold one or two gallons of water. Boil for thirty minutes, squeezing the bag with a wooden spoon every now and then, so that you can extract the maximum amount of ginger from the bag. By the way, don't throw the bag of ginger away, for you can use it again another time, although it will naturally be much weaker. The boiling ginger water should now be poured into the bath water, and you can now immerse and soak yourself in it for twenty to thirty minutes.

This bath is excellent for those suffering from rheumatism, arthritis, muscular cramps, internal congestions or menstruation troubles.

Grass Baths (Tsao Hsi Tsao)

This is a very old Chinese answer to combat what we call the 'water illnesses', which cover rheumatism, arthritis and gout. Get your grass cuttings and place them in a big container and then fill it with water. Boil the grass cuttings and water for thirty minutes then filter the water through a cloth, then pour this grass water into your bath water. Lay in the bath for twenty to thirty minutes, then rinse your body with clean warm water. Then dry yourself and retire immediately to bed. Yes! It is truly wonderful what nature can do.

Of course, there are many more ancient Chinese recommendations, but it is impossible to list them all in a book of this size.

Hip Baths (Tat'ui Hsi Tsao)

There are many old folk who do not like to lie down full-length in a bath, and some are even afraid to do so, and there are many others who because of their particular illness are unable to do so. So they can only sit, and so for these, and also for those who suffer from weak hearts, a hip bath is the ideal way to gain the benefits that heat therapy can give.

There are special hip baths available in the shops, but for those who do not want to buy one, or who cannot afford it, or do not have the space to have one installed, it is possible to use an ordinary bath, though you must ensure that the water only reaches your waistline. Those who cannot stretch their legs out in front of them should put a low stool into the bath and sit on that.

Twenty to thirty minutes is the ideal length of time to stay in a hip bath, so you will need to be able to reach the taps to replenish the bath with extra hot water, or make arrangements for someone to look in every five minutes to do that job for you. Secondly, when having a hip bath always cover the top half of the body with a big towel so you don't catch a cold, and this will also ensure that the upper half of the body can get the benefit of the heat and the steam.

Cabbage Leaves (Pai Tsai Ye)
Use the outside leaves of the cabbage, the ones you would normally throw away, and taking two handfuls of these leaves chop them up, and boil them, with the lid of the pan kept on, for about ten minutes. Then pour the water into the hip bath after having filtered the leaves away. This is good for painful joints, menstruation irregularities, and all forms of cramps. For sterility and leucorrhea, you need to have the water in the hip bath very hot, but make sure that there is always another person present, just in case the heat from the bath water is too overpowering.

Compresses (Ya So)
Compresses or poultices are other heat treatments which cover a reasonably small area of the body, yet they can have varying depths of penetration through the influence that they exert. Some have the qualities to draw out the pain, whilst others can be used to sedate and soothe, or to arouse internal activity.

Onion Poultice (Ts'ung Pa)
Onions should be chopped very finely then placed between two cloths, which, in turn, are then placed on the neck. This will quickly disperse colds, headaches and even earache. This poultice will also stimulate the kidneys when placed in that region. Should a person have heart trouble, the tension can be relieved by placing this poultice on the calves of the legs.

If the onions are heated — and the sautée (stir-fry) method is the best — and then placed in between the cloths, it will greatly aid the circulation, especially in the immediate area on which it is placed, so it is excellent for varicose veins, gout, arthritis, stomach pains and menstruation spasms.

Garlic Poultice (Suan Pa)
Crush or chop the garlic cloves very finely, and then spread evenly

over a soft cloth, to a thickness of about a quarter of an inch, then place another cloth on top. Remember that garlic will burn and/or cause blisters if it is allowed to come in direct contact with the skin. This poultice is excellent for scabies, boils, abscesses and other skin complaints. If the garlic is heated in a frying pan, and then put into a compress, it is very good for breast cancer.

For whooping cough, bronchial and hacking coughs, place the garlic into the cloths, and place them on the bottom of the feet, then slide on an old pair of socks over the top of the compress to hold it steadily in position during the night. This same compress can be used over and over again.

Ginger Compress (Chiang Ya So)
Put four ounces of ginger powder into a small cloth, and then tie the top, and drop it into four pints of boiling water. Simmer for twenty minutes. Now take another cloth and dip it into this ginger water. (It is better to wear rubber gloves at this point.) Then squeeze the cloth out and apply it to the affected area, covering it with another cloth, or a plastic sheet to hold the heat in. Better still, put a hot water bottle on the top. Every three minutes, dip the cloth into the water again, squeeze it out, and apply on the area again. Keep this up for a period of fifteen to twenty minutes.

This is very good for aches and pains in the joints, muscular strains and cramps, kidney troubles, menstruation troubles and cancer (except cancer of the brain). It is also excellent for piles, leprosy, appendicitis, haemorrhoids and sterility.

Cabbage Poultice (Paits'ai Jetien)
Take one leaf from the outside of the cabbage, cut out the thick middle stem, then skim over the whole leaf with a hot electric iron until the surface is as smooth as silk. Then while it is still hot apply it immediately to the painful area of the body. This treatment is ideal for pains from falls or knocks, bruising, rheumatism and muscular tension, and for arthritis and gout and other swellings of the jounts. If you bandage the hot cabbage leaf to the joint or limb, you can go to bed with it strapped to your body, and take it off the next morning. This can be repeated daily to suit the individual and the time that is available.

Soya Bean Curd Poultice (Ta Tou Fu Kaoyao)
Spread the soya bean curd on a cloth to a thickness of about a quarter of an inch, then place it in the required position. Cover

it immediately with another cloth or a plastic sheet. This particular poultice is very good for general aches and pains as well as for inflamed joints or other parts of the body.

If you wish to retain the heat of the poultice or compress over a long period of time, place a hot water bottle on top of the cloth. If you wish, this poultice can be left on all night by simply bandaging it to the affected area.

Hot Water Bottles (Je Shui P'ing)
This can always be used to relax the muscles in a specific part of the body, and it will also ease many forms of pain, including menstrual spasms. It will also aid the general circulation of the blood within the body, and for this reason it is excellent when placed under the soles of the feet of the arthritic sufferer. If it causes perspiration, then the hot water bottle is doing its job, and it is good for the person concerned.

Herbs (Tsao)
There are literally hundreds of excellent herbs that are used in this particular section of the Chinese arts, and each one has its own specific values and uses. This great interest in natural healing methods has never been lost to the Chinese, and thank goodness, interest in the West, is again getting stronger as every day goes by. Yes! The old creates the foundations of the new. In China, we have an old saying: 'If you want to advance, the surest way is to take one pace forward and two steps back.'

Other Methods of Thermogenesis
In addition to the other methods already cited, there are two other methods of applying heat to areas of the body with the object of speeding up the processes of recovery. Both have been used from very ancient times to the present day.

The first method is by the use of a brass ladle into which is laid a copper wire mesh. On top of the mesh are laid some dried leaves of the mugwort plant, which are then ignited. These leaves burn very slowly, but as soon as the bowl of the brass ladle begins to get warm, a piece of cotton gauze or a thin layer of cloth is placed over the affected part of the body, and the base of the ladle is then rubbed gently on the gauze or the cloth so that the heat slowly penetrates through. It is then that the affected area of the body will feel the comfort and the soothing effect of this particular heat treatment.

Now to the second method. Do any of you remember the old-fashioned bed-warmer that was once very common in the West, that looked like a straight-sided frying pan with a lid on the top? Well, in China we have something similar but very much smaller in size. The bowl is no bigger than the palm of the hand, and it has a hinged lid. This is filled with warm ashes from the fire, and again covering the area of the body with a thin cloth or gauze, we can then apply the heat treatment in the same way as we did with the ladle. Both are still used extensively in Chinese heat treatments.

Finally, we come to cold compresses. It may seem strange that our section on thermogenesis includes the use of cold water and ice packs, but the theory and the basic principles behind this practice are still the underlying foundations created by Yin and Yang. Heat, which is Yang, can be exerted or absorbed inwardly (Yin), but the body (Yin), through rejection or compulsion, can throw it in an outward direction (Yang), and it is in this latter case that cold compresses can be used to help lower the temperature levels and also create internal restriction.

Chapter 8

Anmo — Taoist Massage

When you feel the cold, there is a natural tendency to try to create warmth by rubbing certain areas of your skin, such as your hands or arms, to cause the required friction. Similarly, if you have a painful joint, then it is an automatic reflex action to give it a rub or even exercise it in some way. Then again, if you pull a muscle, then it is completely natural for you to try and ease the tension by manipulating the affected section of your body. Such automatic reactions are natural to all mankind, and they do help you to eradicate such things as cold, pain and stress of any kind, at any time, even though you may have no knowledge of massage whatsoever.

In China, however, remedial massage has been practised for literally thousands of years, for it was the 'Sons of Reflected Light' (Fankuang Tzu) who taught us how to energize or sedate the body through the correct use of the hands. Having learnt the depth of this art it was a natural step to separate certain sections for further research, and that is why there came into being the techniques of acupressure (Tien Chen) and then finally acupuncture (Hsia Chen Pien). This deep research led to the discovery and utilization of the energy channels, which are known today as the meridian lines, and it was found that it was possible to stimulate or soothe, depending on the particular technique or point used, certain areas on the surface of the skin, which in turn, could convey certain effects to the internal parts of the body. So these arts also had a completely natural Yin and Yang application.

Whilst the Chinese Taoist systems of massages are very simple, they are also extremely effective, and they have proved themselves over and over again as a very dynamic form of therapeutics, and, as such, have well established themselves in the healthy arts of China.

Taoist massage (Anmo) has been taught in Chinese medical schools over many centuries, but unfortunately it did decline drastically during the Sung Period (960-1276), so much so that it took a very long time before it got back into the curriculum of the medical profession that existed during that period. However, once it had re-established itself, it was not long before it was again being used in conjunction with all the other methods of treatment. Today it is taught as a completely separate art, and it has the distinct advantage that it can be used entirely on its own, without the use of any other treatments, and yet it can equally harmonize with Ch'ang Ming (Taoist long life health diet), and also with Ts'ao Yao (herbal therapy), and in so doing it creates a balance of the Yin and Yang, which in this case, provides internal and external therapy at the same time, so the period of recuperation is accelerated.

It can break down the harmful effects of fatty tissue, strengthen muscular sinews, relieve cramps and spasms, and help in cases of rheumatism, osteo- and rheumatoid arthritis, chronic back troubles, paralysis of the nerves, and multiple sclerosis. It can ease the tension of stiff joints, increase the body resistance to colds, fevers, chills, coughing and asthma, as well as combating diarrhoea and constipation, indigestion, ulcers, anuria and hernia. It will eradicate headaches, migraines and facial paralysis, and, depending on the techniques that are used, it will sedate or stimulate the flow of Ch'i (internal energy) along the lines of the meridians to the various organs of the body. It can also have similar effects on the circulation of the blood, and also on the respiratory system.

In view of the foregoing it can be fully appreciated that Anmo is also excellent for the whole digestive and bowel system, helping the body to become generally healthier and more active, through the toning up of the muscles and tissues. And in doing all this, it is enabling the body to combat all kinds of internal diseases and infections. In so doing, it will gain greater strength and better health to withstand external cold, excessive heat and bacteria. That is why it is now widely and commonly used throughout China for the treatment of children, adults, the very old and the sick.

It is wonderful to know that not only has Taoist massage (Anmo) taken its rightful place within the medical profession of China, but that the medical professions and alternative medicine groups outside of China have taken up this very ancient art in a big way. Specialized classes are now being held in England, Wales, France, Germany and Holland, but enquiries are pouring in from all over the world, from people whose one aim in life is to help others to overcome the handicaps of modern society.

The Techniques

Taoist massage (Anmo) falls into two main groups, and like all things connected with the Chinese Taoist philosophical outlook, each group conforms to the principles of the Tao, abiding by the dualism of Yin and Yang, which in turn encompasses the five statutes of the natural elements (Wu Hsing). These groups and the systems which fall within the scope of their remedial massage are as follows:

Stimulation (Yang) techniques
1. Grasping.
2. Kneading.
3. Pinch-pull.
4. Rubbing.
5. Tapping.

Sedation (Yin) techniques
1. Pressing.
2. Rotating.
3. Rolling.
4. Wiping and scraping.
5. Pushing.

It may come as a surprise to you to see only these few techniques listed above, but bear in mind that each system has many individual sections. For instance, Rubbing has six different techniques, all of which have very specific jobs to do. Bear in mind, too, that not only are they extremely beneficial on their own, but, when coupled with the dietary and herbal sections of the Taoist arts, their success rate has been almost unbelievable in combating many serious illnesses.

Anyone wishing to practise Anmo, however, should first of all learn the system of diagnosis, both internal and external. Secondly, a good knowledge of the Ch'i energy that is constantly flowing through the meridian lines of the body, the direction of the flow, and the points or centres along the meridians, should all be studied diligently. Thirdly, it is extremely important to ensure that you exercise your fingers, hands, wrists and arms as often as you can. The object is not to make them stronger and harder, but to make them more supple and more flexible.

Once you start to practise our Taoist massage on yourself, or even amongst your friends, you will fully appreciate how important it is to execute a few daily exercises that will help to strengthen your fingers, especially your index and middle fingers, and also the thumbs of both hands (see Fig. 3). You can do this by the simple expedient of flexing them daily for at least two or three minutes, and then firmly pressing them down onto a table or any other hard surface for another two minutes. You can also press the fingers and thumbs of both hands against each other during the course of each day, for further light exercising.

The wrists should be flexed regularly both forwards and backwards, and you should try and strengthen your grip by making a fist with your hands and gripping as tight as you can. When I myself was first learning the arts, I used to carry two very small rubber balls in my pockets, and when the opportunity permitted, I used to squeeze them as hard as possible, with alternate hands, in time with my steps as I walked along the street. It is important, as you will find out, to practise a few simple exercises in the early stages, as often as you can, at least three to four times daily.

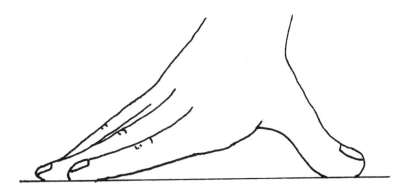

Fig. 3   Exercising the thumb.

Now try exercising your fingers and thumbs by pressing one hand against the other, as shown in Fig. 4.

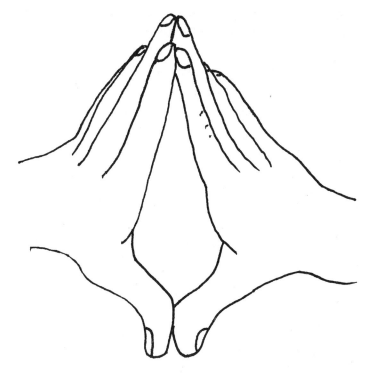

Fig. 4   Finger exercise no. 1.

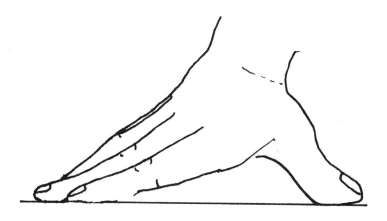

Fig. 5   Finger exercise no. 2.

Fig. 5 shows how you can press firmly down on a hard surface, to help strengthen the units of your hand; but don't overdo it at first.

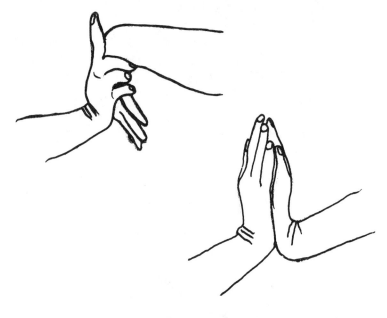

Fig. 6 Exercising the wrist.

Now bend the wrist forward and back (see Fig. 6).

In addition to these exercises, don't forget to grip your hands into very tight fists as often as you can, for you need very strong yet flexible hands when having to massage people for any length of time. In ancient China, students used to exercise their hands and wrists by practising their massage techniques on sacks filled with grain or rice, and trying to dehusk the grain or rice with their bare hands was a very hard yet effective way to strengthen the fingers, thumbs and palms.

An important point to remember in our Taoist massage, is that it is not just a matter of moving muscles and ligaments to relieve tension, and just because a person's back happens to ache, it does not necessarily mean that you have to massage that particular spot. You have to be absolutely certain that the point or area of the body that you intend to massage is the right one for the particular job in hand, and that the direction of massage will ensure that it will change the distribution and equilibrium of the Ch'i energy, and also that the organ of the body is the correct one for that particular part or area. In other words, everything you do must conform entirely to the requirements of the body and must be in accord with the principles of Yin and Yang.

Chinese massage, then, is not a haphazard affair, but a very precise art which has a deep understanding of the human body and the natural laws of the universe as laid down by the Tao. For instance, if there is a Yin aspect in the body, which will show a deficiency of energy, sluggishness, low activity, lethargy, and a fluctuation of internal rhythm, then it will have to be countered by a Yang influence, which in Taoist massage is accomplished through techniques of stimulation. Conversely, the Yang aspect in the human body will reflect excess energy, increased activity, pain of all kinds, and a very strong flow of energy rhythm. The only way that this can be tackled with confidence is through the use of a Yin application, which simply means that the overworked systems must be soothed and sedated.

Whilst the range of Taoist massage techniques is wide, and very comprehensive, it is possible to give an outline of the main sections:

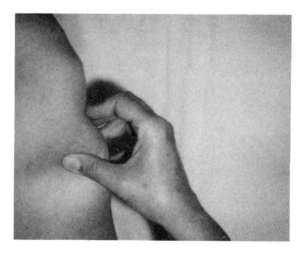

Grasping (Chua-Fa) — Fig. 7
The individual muscle cords on the neck and shoulders, under the arms, on the sides of the body, the front of the intestines and bladder, the buttocks and most parts of the legs, can be gripped between the thumb and fingers. Then the muscle cords can be lifted, shaken or vibrated, which will tone and stimulate.

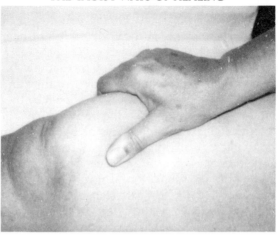

Kneading (Jou-Fa) — Fig. 8
This is suitable for the face, abdomen, arms and the lower extremities of the body, and can also be used around the area of a swelling or a tumour. It is applied by using the heel of the palm, and at the same time holding the flesh with the fingers to form a base. This action is very similar to kneading the dough when making bread.

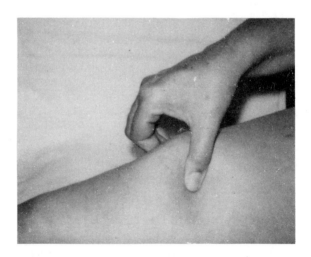

Pinch-pull (Chia-La-Fa) — Fig. 9
The skin and/or the muscle cords are gripped between the thumb and fingers. The skin or cord is then pulled until it actually pops

out of the grip or pinch. The pinch is always executed away from the body, and it can be used on all parts of the face, neck and body. The tenacity of the pinch can be gentle, medium or strong, depending upon the area of the body that is to be massaged and the person involved, but even the strongest pinch should not bring a cry of anguish from the patient.

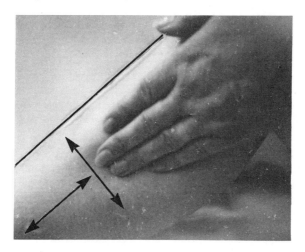

Rubbing (Ts'uo-Fa) — Fig. 10
This method is suitable for all parts of the body, including the neck and face. It is executed with the fingers, the ball of the thumb or the whole hand, in a quick motion and always in two directions, either forward and back, or sideways to the left and then right (or vice versa). With adults only, the skin or the cords can be held between the two palms and a forward and back motion applied.

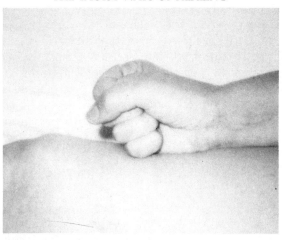

Tapping (P'ai-Fa) — Fig. 11
This particular group of techniques can be used with considerable variation in the degree of force that is applied, and can be executed directly onto the person's skin or indirectly by using the back of your own hand. It is absolutely forbidden, however, to use any of these techniques on young children.

The above five main sections cover the stimulation of the whole muscular system (Hsingfen) and they are all Yang techniques. Now we come to the sedation (Ch'en Ching) methods which completely oppose the above, because they are all Yin techniques.

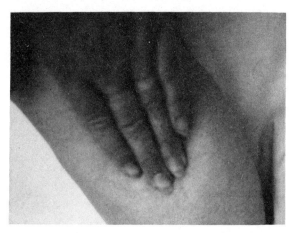

Pushing (T'ui-fa) — Fig. 12
This is a simple method, for all one has to do is to push along the

surface of the skin, with a firm and positive action but always in a vertical direction. For this system we can use either the ball of the thumb, the tips of the fingers, or the heel of the palm, and the pressure can be applied to the neck, chest, abdomen, lumbar region or any of the limbs.

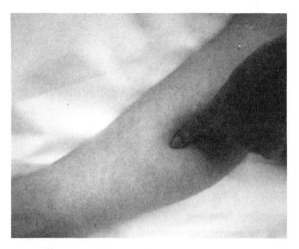

Pressing (Ya-Fa) — *Fig. 13*
This involves the greatest range of areas of the whole body in which Taoist massage is practised, and so great is its volume of work that the Old Masters of this art eventually found it necessary to separate it, and make it a complete art within itself. Today it is called Tien Chen (spot pressing, or acupressure). It is dealt with fully in Chapter 9.

Pressing can be accomplished by the use of one finger, or the ball of the thumb, or the use of all the fingertips simultaneously, or even the whole hand. The degree of pressure can vary according to the area being massaged, and it can be gentle, moderate or strong. It can be applied to all parts of the head, neck, limbs and trunk.

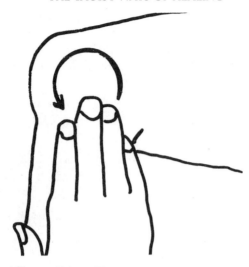

Rotating (Chuan-Fa) — Fig. 14
These techniques are admirably suitable for all the body joints, for swellings and for tumours. The edge of the thumb or the tips of the fingers are used in a movement which is circular in its flow around all the joints, and around any kind of swelling or tumour. It is especially useful on the rib cage and the abdomen as well.

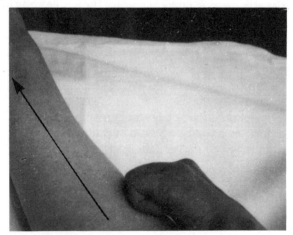

Rolling (Kunpao-Fa) — Fig. 15
Because of the power of this technique it is used only on the shoulder, the back, the waist, the buttocks and the legs. It is done by using the back of the hand or the back of the fist, very gently to start with, but then slowly increasing the power and the pressure during the execution.

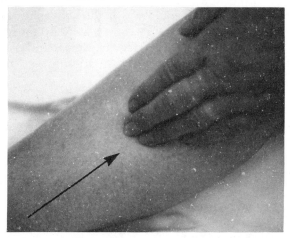

Wiping and Scraping (Ts'a-Fa) — Fig. 16
Both of these methods can be used on most part of the body but
only wiping is used on the face. Scraping is never used on children
nor on people with delicate or very dry skins. The pressure applied
normally is gentle at first, but it can be increased if necessary.

Anyone who intends to practise Taoist massage (Anmo) regularly,
should remember these three very important rules:

1. Always exercise your thumbs, fingers and wrists regularly, to
   make them both subtle and strong, otherwise you will find
   that you become very fatigued, both mentally and physically.
2. Always smear a little oil or cream on the area of the patient's
   body where treatment is to be given, ensuring that the oil or
   cream that is used is soluble to the human body.
3. Never massage the area where the patient feels pain.

The *Nei Ching* mentions the benefits of Anmo on many occasions.
Here are a few of its recommendations:

1. People in the centre of China have the tendency to suffer from
   paralysis, colds, chills and fevers, and these can be combated
   easily by the use of Anmo, Tao Yin (Taoist respiration therapy)
   K'ai Men (Taoist Chi Kung, sometimes referred to as Taoist
   yoga) and T'ai Chi Ch'uan (The Supreme Ultimate).
2. Should circulation in the arteries and veins cease due to shock
   or nervous complaints, and thereby the sensitivity of feel
   disappears, and numbness within the body arises, then it is
   essential that herbal therapy (Ts'ao Yao) and massage (Anmo)
   is used to cure these illnesses.

3. When there is insufficient energy in the body, one must first feel with the hand to trace the circuit, and also the high and low levels within the system. Having thus found out where there is sufficient and also where there is insufficient, then one must apply Anmo accordingly.

The External Aspect (Yang)
This covers the muscular system and the joints of the body, and it has both Yin and Yang techniques. In the case of physical fatigue, numbness or a very weak muscular system, then it is important to apply stimulation (Yang) techniques, and where there is pain, stress or strain in the physical aspect then obviously sedation (Yin) techniques must be used.

The Internal Aspect (Yin)
These are methods which most people in the Western world have found difficult to understand and fully appreciate at first, yet the results have been proved, over thousands of years, to be absolutely dynamic.

Stimulation (Yang)
This is to fully activate the energy levels within any of the twelve organs and the main eight centres of the human body. This enables the masseur (Anmo Shih) or masseuse (Anmo Nu) to boost the energy reserves during low or run-down periods, and to combat the fatigue that accompanies them in the Yin times of the year.

Sedation (Yin)
Amazing though it may seem, this puts into the hands of the practitioner the ability to sedate areas of the body which are giving pain caused through sickness and disease. In the majority of cases, complete cures can be affected by the simple expedient of being able to combat the source of the trouble, whether it started in the organs of the body or not. Very good examples of the dynamic potential of this art are that migraine can be stopped completely within twenty-four hours, and a stiff neck can be eradicated within a few seconds.

What is the first thing you do when you go outside in winter and feel the impact of the cold atmostphere hitting your skin? Let me remind you. You either start to rub your hands together, or you slap them to increase the circulation in your palms and fingers. This is completely natural. You will therefore fully appreciate why the Taoist looked into this very simple yet very natural action to see if it had any connection with Anmo. Naturally it did, for rubbing is one of the many techniques involved, but did it have any effect on the body and the organs?

The connection between Anmo and the organs became more apparent when the flow of energy through the meridian channels was discovered, and through this it was realized that by massaging certain parts of the hands, feet and body, the practitioner could also gain access to the organs. So, in cold weather, if you want to stimulate your circulation and get warm faster, then all you have to do is to utilize a very simple Chinese Taoist massage technique.

If you are going to rub your right hand, then put your right palm facing towards you, then with the fingers of your left hand rub your right palm facing towards you, then with the fingers of your left hand rub your right palm and fingers in an anti-clockwise direction. If you rub your left hand then rub it with your right hand in a clockwise direction, and you will really feel the difference that it makes not only in your hands and arms but also inside your body. Of course, you can also rub both hands at the same time, by a palm-to-palm contact, but check that you rotate them in the correct direction.

This simple technique will show you that Anmo can be practised by all those who allow themselves the opportunity of understanding the techniques and principles laid down by our very ancient ancestors in China, and of developing a greater awareness of everything that concerns ourselves.

Chapter 9

Tien Chen — Acupressure

Tien Chen is another very ancient art of China, and one which is the forerunner of Hsia Chen Pien (acupuncture). It was realized that many of the energy centres along the lines of meridians lay fairly close to the surface of the skin, and therefore it did not need a deep instrument to get at them, but only the pressure of a finger or thumb. After thousands of years of testing it was realized that although excellent results were obtained by this system of spot pressing, it needed to be a little more precise in its application and so the ancients introduced using the tips of their fingernails as well as the tip of a blunt instrument.

So whereas Hsia Chen Pien has always used a variety of needles for its work along the meridian channels, the Tien Chen practitioner needs only some of the tools of the human body to execute the various techniques employed in his art. In conformity with the 'Five Elements' (Wu Hsing), these are:

1. The tip of the thumb.
2. The tip of the index finger.
3. The second knuckle of the middle finger.
4. The nail of the thumb or index finger.
5. Yuan Chen — the round-headed needle.

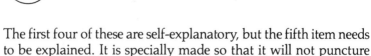

The first four of these are self-explanatory, but the fifth item needs to be explained. It is specially made so that it will not puncture the skin when a downward pressure is exerted, yet its head must not cover too large an area when placed on the skin. It is small enough to be carried at all times in the pocket, so that it is handy in case of emergencies. An erasure pencil with the rubber rounded off at the end is just as good, and because the rubber gives slightly it can be used on adults and children alike.

Even with Tien Chen there are two aims to be obtained; sedation and stimulation. Sedation is gained by applying pressure gradually until a heavy pressure is reached. It is then maintained for ten or fifteen seconds. For stimulation, the pressure is applied rapidly to the required depth, and released just as quickly, then applied again and released, and this may be continued for thirty seconds.

Remember that the majority of cases that you will come up against involve pain, and you must therefore 'drain for pain', or in other words you must sedate. However, remember that when you treat pain you are simply removing a symptom, though in many cases the work you have done will eradicate the cause, leaving the body to carry on its own work internally completely unhindered.

Draining or sedating, however, also takes away a certain amount of the person's vitality power of Ch'i energy, and this commodity is too precious to be wasted, as it is the lifeline of the body. We must take steps to ensure that it is not wasted. For example, if the pain were at one end of the meridian, in the chest, we could place moxa or other heat treatment at the other end of the meridian, in the region of the thumb. This has a twofold benefit; (1) it draws the energy away from the painful area, and (2) external heat brings in external energy, so no energy is wasted within the person.

Another typical example of this is the fever or influenza, and we have a saying in China: 'Keep the head cool, the feet hot and the centre just right.' So you put cold compresses on the forehead to combat the fever, which acts as a form of sedation; a hot water bottle under the feet, which brings in external energy; and a bowl of warm vegetable soup to keep the centre of the body just right.

Through pulse study you may find an indication that there is a deficiency in one of the other meridians, which is not being affected by the pain, so it is possible to drain or sedate the excess of energy from the painful area of a particular meridian, and put it into the meridian that is deficient. By doing so, you have created the perfect balance between the Yang and Yin aspects of the two meridians, and this is working perfectly to the order of the universe.

It is impossible in a book of this size to put down every illness and the numerous points of the meridians that apply to each one; there are 400 meridian points on the head alone. However, I have listed quite a number of them, together with the meridians and the meridian points for each complaint, and you can select one or two to use for the person who needs help, and you can choose the ones that you wish to sedate or stimulate.

Angina pectoris
Gall Bladder 20, 21, 44
Bladder 64
Lung 1, 2, 4
Circulation 5, 6

Arteriosclerosis
Gall Bladder 31, 39
Stomach 36
Bladder 60, 62
Circulation 8
Liver 2, 4

Arthritis
Heart 4
Triple Heater 4, 5, 12
Small Intestine 4, 9
Bladder 54, 60, 61, 67
Kidney 10
Gall Bladder, 33, 34, 38
Stomach, 35, 37, 38, 42

Bronchitis
Circulation 2, 3
Lung 1, 3, 5
Large Intestine 8
Stomach 10
Conception 23

Constipation
Large Intestine 2
Triple Heater 6
Bladder 27, 28, 30, 32, 33, 34, 48, 50, 52, 56
Kidney 3, 4, 8, 15, 16
Liver 1, 2
Gall Bladder 34

Depression
Heart 9
Large Intestine 4, 11
Spleen 6

Diabetes
Triple Heater 4
Kidney 2
Liver 1, 2
Conception 24

Epilepsy
Triple Heater 12
Small Intestine 2, 3, 5
Bladder 53, 58, 61, 63, 64
Conception 24
Stomach 41, 42

Headache
Circulation 7
Lung 7, 10
Small Intestine 1, 4, 7
Bladder 10, 60, 62, 65, 66, 67
Gall Bladder 44
Stomach 2, 36, 40, 41

Laryngitis
Large Intestine 1, 2
Bladder 11, 12, 13
Kidney 3, 7

Rheumatism
Lung 3
Large Intestine 12, 13
Triple Heater 4, 12
Bladder 58
Gall Bladder 33, 42
Stomach 41

Tonsillitis
Stomach 10, 38, 39, 45
Gall Bladder 38, 39
Kidney 1, 2, 6
Triple Heater 1, 2, 3
Large Intestine 1, 2, 3, 4, 5, 6, 7, 11

Toothache
Lung 7
Heart 3
Large intestine 1, 3, 4, 6, 10
Triple Heater 5, 8, 9
Gall Bladder 2

Vomiting
Lung 3, 4, 8
Triple Heater 1, 6
Small Intestine 4
Kidney 2, 3, 4
Spleen 3, 4, 5

Remember that it is important that you always rebalance the system after treatment, especially when sedating, and there are two meridian points well worth remembering which will help you tone up the system after you have drained it. These are: Large Intestine 4, which, when vibrated to stimulate, will aid the upper part of the body; and Bladder 60, which will help to recover some of the energy for the lower part of the body.

Chapter 10

Hsia Chen Pien — Acupuncture

Hsia Chen Pien is the Chinese name for acupuncture, which is derived from Latin, and means 'to puncture with a needle'. It is an art that is truly unique to the Chinese, and which has become a part of their heritage, through the knowledge imparted to them by the 'Sons of Reflected Light'.

Originally, only stone needles were used for this work, but today they are made of gold, silver and stainless steel. All of them are made in a variety of lengths, the shortest being half an inch long, and the longest up to three inches. More publicity has been given to this art over the last few years, and more and more of the general public are becoming aware of it. Therapy is effected through the use and manipulation of the needles, which have the tendency to influence, stimulate, sedate and activate, and to eradicate the causes of many forms of sickness, helping to achieve internal harmony, and thereby enabling the body to fight its way back to good health.

But what are the underlying principles of this art, and what do we have to know and eventually accomplish? For we cannot utilize Hsia Chen Pien to heal others unless we have this knowledge and the skills to apply it.

The natural internal energy of the body (Sheng Ch'i or just 'Ch'i'), is sometimes referred to as the 'vitality force', was passed on to you whilst you were still in your mother's uterus, and when you were born it became your responsibility to ensure that its level remained at a constant state to give yourself good health. This energy should be a part of every organ and every cell in the tissue of your body. It is the natural manifestation, activation, flow and rhythm of it that enables it to conform to the universal laws, and it is through the nutritional value of the food that we eat, and our respiration, that cultivation of this energy is possible.

Due to bad eating and drinking habits and poor breathing

tendencies, however, this energy (Ch'i) slowly becomes depleted, and illness becomes a reality. It can also go the other way: through these same bad habits an excess can be built up so that another imbalance is created, and again sickness rears its ugly head. If there is a complete lack of energy then cancer or death is not far away.

In conformity to the principles of the Five Elements (Wu Hsing), Sheng Ch'i has five stages:

1. Greater Yang, when you are still in your mother's womb.
2. Lesser Yang, from infancy to adolescence.
3. Central, when you are mature and fully grown, and your energy settles down to its natural healthy level.
4. Lesser Yin, your later years, when deterioration of your internal energy starts to take place.
5. Greater Yin, when all energy disappears and death results.

You will have noticed that this is not based on a specific total or number of years, because you can create an imbalance at any time within your own system, and if you don't correct it in time and restore it to its natural healthy level, then you will automatically enter into stage 4, which is the stage of deterioration, and thereby shorten your own lifespan.

The practitioner of Hsai Chen Pien must be able to recognize the illness or disease through his skill in the five sections of diagnosis, and in many instances, if the patient comes to him in time, he can combat a complaint long before any symptom of the illness can manifest itself, and thereby he can actually prevent it at its source. So he finds the energy imbalance and the organ or organs that are involved, then through his work he endeavours to restore the energy to its correct level by the insertion of the needles.

The Meridians

Ch'i circulates through our body system along well-established channels, which are called meridians (Ching), which link the meridian points or spots, so that they form a definite pattern of lines, each of which is associated with a specific organ of the body and takes the name of that organ. The existence of the meridians and their points has been repeatedly questioned by many Western doctors, who often consider the Chinese ancient therapy doctor to be a quack. Many countries, however, such as Japan, Russia and France, have themselves proved the scientific value of this very ancient art. This has been facilitated by the modern usage of very highly electro-sensitive instruments, which have proved that the ancient Chinese were absolutely right.

Ch'i energy and its flow are closely associated with the autonomic nervous system, which is linked to every organ and to all parts of the anatomy, including the skin tissue and glands. It is the sedation or activation of the meridians and their points that affects the flow of Ch'i, either by slowing it down, or by giving it a boost so that the benefits may be felt and recorded by the autonomic nervous system, which will, in turn, affect specific areas of the organs or various parts of the body.

There are twelve meridians or channels, ten of which are connected to specific organs, the other two being related to internal body activity. These twelve meridians are known as bilateral as they have a uniformity of lines on both sides of the body, and Ch'i energy is constantly flowing along them in a specific direction. These meridians and the direction of flow are as follows:

Organ	Yin or Yang	Direction of Ch'i
Heart	Yin	Centrifugal
Small Intestine	Yang	Centripetal
Liver	Yin	Centripetal
Gall Bladder	Yang	Centrifugal
Spleen/Pancreas	Yin	Centripetal
Stomach	Yang	Centrifugal
Lungs	Yin	Centrifugal
Large Intestine	Yang	Centripetal
Kidneys	Yin	Centripetal
Urinary Bladder	Yang	Centrifugal
Heart Circulation	Yin	Centrifugal
Triple Heater	Yang	Centripetal

We know that each Yin organ is paired off with a specific Yang organ, and the direction of energy will flow along one meridian until it reaches the extreme limits of the limb, and then it will flow along the path of the meridian to which it is paired. This is why we have two different directions of flow with each pair of organs, as you may have noticed above.

The Heart Circulation, sometimes referred to as the Controller of the Heart or Heart Governor, is involved in the complete circulation of the blood, and the energy that is within the blood throughout the whole body. The Triple Heater, sometimes called the Three Burning Spheres, controls the chemical activity within the body. In addition to this, however, it also has other important jobs to do, for it also regulates and adjusts body temperature changes, and transfers heat and Ch'i energy from one area to another. However, neither Heart Circulation nor Triple Heater are 'organs' in the strict technical sense of the word.

All of the Yin meridians have their lines or paths running on the inside of the arms or the legs, whilst the Yang meridians run along the outside of these same limbs. Ch'i energy circulates through the entire body within a twenty-four-hour period, with each organ having a two-hour minimum period of activity, and a two-hour minimum period of flow, so even our energies conform to the Yin and Yang principles.

However, if the Ch'i flowing through the body is slowed down or restricted by some internal blockage, or is made to flow faster than normal through an external influence, or there is extra energy in the system, then the organism of the body is thrown out of balance, and this can result in sickness.

It is on this understanding that the acupuncturist can give tonification to the organ or organs that have low energy levels, or even sedate them if they are overactive, and through this Yin and Yang application, harmony can be restored once again within the organism of the body.

Peak Periods

So accurate have the Chinese studies in the art of Hsia Chen Pien been, that they can tell when the high and low energy levels will take place in the years ahead, the seasons, the days and the hours. So let us look at the last of these and understand the two-hour peak period of each of the twelve meridians and their connected organs.

A.M.

Time	Yin/Yang	Organ
1 to 3 a.m.	Yin	Liver
3 to 5 a.m.	Yin	Lungs
5 to 7 a.m.	Yang	Large Intestine
7 to 9 a.m.	Yang	Stomach
9 to 11 a.m.	Yin	Spleen/Pancreas
11 a.m. to 1 p.m.	Yin	Heart

P.M.

Time	Yin/Yang	Organ
1 to 3 p.m.	Yang	Small Intestine
3 to 5 p.m.	Yang	Bladder
5 to 7 p.m.	Yin	Kidneys
7 to 9 p.m.	Yin	Heart Circulation
9 to 11 p.m.	Yang	Triple Heater
11 p.m. to 1 a.m.	Yang	Gall Bladder

Bear in mind that if the Liver, for instance, is working at its peak between one and three o'clock in the morning, then it will be at its lowest ebb or weakest period between one and three o'clock in the afternoon. It has been found that an excess energy complaint within an organ is more responsive to treatment during the peak periods of activity, so treatment would commence just a short time before maximum activity starts. In the case of those suffering from low energy or weak periods, then the ideal time to start the treatment would be immediately after the peak period has ended.

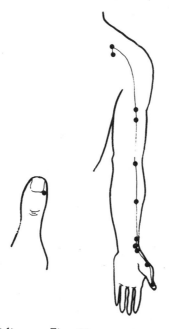

The Lung Meridian — Fig. 17
The Lung meridian (Yin) is indirectly connected to the Large Intestine meridian (Yang) and sends its energy to it in a centrifugal

motion. It has eleven points (on each arm), four of which are forbidden to moxa and to other forms of heat treatment. These four points are Nos. 3, 8, 10 and 11.

This meridian covers the disorders of the respiratory system, such as asthma, bronchitis, coughs, inflammation of the lungs, intermittent and tropical fever, fear and anxiety neurosis, facial paralysis, articular rheumatism, and vertigo.

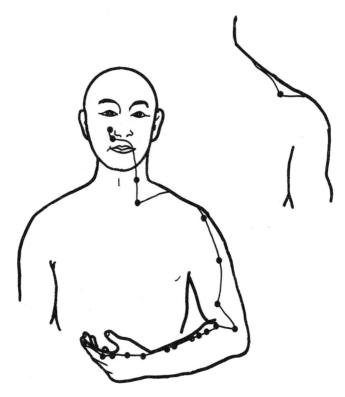

The Large Intestine Meridian — Fig. 18
The Large Intestine meridian (Yang) receives its energy from the Lung meridian, and in turn, it transmits Ch'i force to the Stomach meridian (Yang).

This meridian starts on the index finger at the root of the nail, but slightly towards the thumb. It then runs externally up the arm, ventral side to the clavicle, then slightly over the shoulder, and then back to the upper breastbone, then via the lower jawbone and the corner of the mouth (where it influences the lower lip), then to the other side of the nostril to the depression known as

the nasogenion fold. There are twenty points (on each arm), three
of which are banned to moxa and other heat treatments, and these
points are Nos. 13, 19 and 20.

Many of the throat, mouth and nose complaints can be attributed
to the Large Intestine, such as dry throat, parched lips, inflamed
tongue, tonsillitis, toothache, swollen jaws, catarrh, bronchitis,
absent sense of smell, as well as headaches, apoplexy, depressions,
fear and frights in children, polyps of the nose, and poor eyesight.

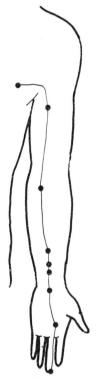

The Heart Circulation Meridian — Fig. 19
This meridian obtains its Ch'i energy from the Kidney meridian,
and it starts halfway between the nipple and the armpit, travelling
along the inside of the arm, and finishing its journey on the inside
of the tip of the middle finger, at the root of the nail.

The Heart Circulation meridian, sometimes called the Heart
Governor, is Yin, and it runs in a centrifugal direction. There are
no points along this meridian that are banned to moxa or heat
treatment. It has a total of nine meridian points (eighteen if you
count both arms).

The West does not recognize this particular system as an organ, and technically it is not, but the Chinese in their ancient wisdom, appreciated that an organ does not necessarily have to be in one piece to be effective, so they considered the whole vascular system to be an organ within itself. It covers the arteries, veins and capillaries, which deal with the circulation of fluids in the body, haemorrhages, gastritis, insufficient milk in the breasts, female sterility, and inflammation of the heart.

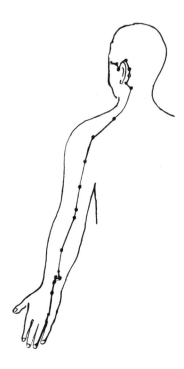

The Triple Heater Meridian — Fig. 20
This is another organ not recognized in the West, and we agree, it is a tough one to imagine. The Chinese saw it as being composed of three sections: respiration energy; the regulating of the digestive system; and the control of the processes of the urogenital and sex organs, including the chemical changes within the complete system. It is Yang and receives its Ch'i energy from the Heart Circulation meridian, and in turn, passes on the surplus to the Gall Bladder meridian. The Ch'i flows in a centripetal direction, from the little finger edge of your ring finger nail and runs up the outside of the

arm, to the rear of the shoulder, then round the back of the ear, circles up and down round the ear, then passes to the joint of the lower jawbone, and out to the temple at the corner of the eye. It has a total of twenty-three points, or forty-six if you count both arms.

It covers a very wide range of illnesses, including contracted lips, toothache, neuralgia, vertigo, apoplexy, cerebral congestions, deafness, epilepsy, gingivitis, nephritis, and paralysis and spasms in the arms and neck.

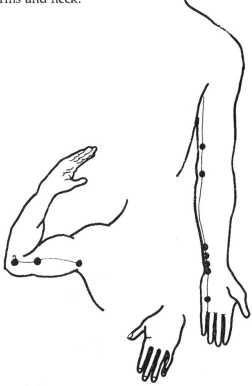

The Heart Meridian — Fig. 21
The Heart meridian (Yin) get its Ch'i energy from the Spleen meridian, and in turn, passes this energy, which flows in a centrifugal motion, on to the Small Intestine. It has a total of nine points on each arm, making a total of eighteen overall.

The first point is situated at the every top of the arm in the apex of the axilla, and it runs down the inside of the arm, and then on to the inside edge of the little finger to the final point, which is near to the fingernail fold.

This meridian is of great value in combatting a number of psychologically and emotionally caused stresses, as well as other physical illnesses such as nervous anxiety, hysteria, psychopathy, melancholy, depressions, neuralgia of the arm and face, pulmonary tuberculosis, leucorrhoea, epistaxis, arthritis in the elbow, cold sensations in the elbow, wrist and arm, vulvar pruritis, endocarditis, adenopathy, metrorrhagia, and general weaknesses caused by fevers and influenza. It is also excellent for those who suffer from insomnia.

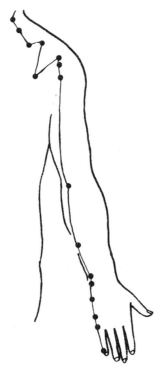

The Small Intestine Meridian — Fig. 22
The Small Intestine meridian is Yang and its receives its Ch'i energy from the Heart meridian, and transmits it in a centripetal direction from the outer edge of the little finger's nail root, up the exterior side of the arm to the back of the shoulder joint, over the shoulder blade, up the side of the neck, to the upper part of the lower jaw bone, out to the centre of the cheek, then back to a point in front of the ear. It has nineteen points, thirty-eight for both arms.

Overactiveness or weakness in the state of this meridian will indicate a wide range of diseases and sickness, including swollen throat, tonsillitis, coughs, stiff neck, oedema, epilepsy, coryza, neuralgia, gingivitis, tinnitus, pneumonia, aphonia, toothache, fever, weak eyesight, mastitis, madness, paralysis of the arm, fear and apprehension in children, anal fistula, pleurisy, sternal pains and agalactia.

It has only two points which are forbidden to heat treatment.

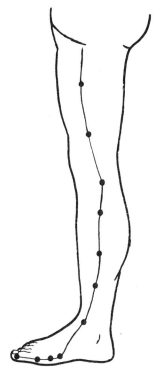

The Spleen Meridian — Fig. 23

This meridian obtains its energy from the Stomach meridian, and it is Yin. It directs its energy in a centripetal direction of flow, and then eventually it passes it on to the Heart meridian. It has twenty-one points on each leg, with three points banned for heat treatment.

This meridian starts on the outside of the nail fold of the big toe, then runs directly back to halfway along the foot, and up the outside of the leg, through the groin to a point just below the navel, then up to the second intercostal space, from where it drops down to the sixth intercostal space almost under the armpit.

It covers a vast range of disturbances — all diseases of the genital organs of both sexes, abdominal swelling and pain, fever and fatigue, buttock pains, menorrhagia, orchitis, influenza, dyspnoea, dysuria, haemorrhoids, lumbago, vomiting, ascites, hyperacidity and cardiac pain.

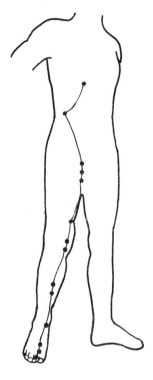

The Liver Meridian — Fig. 24
The Liver meridian is another Yin character for it flows in a centripetal direction, and obtains its Ch'i energy from the Gall Bladder meridian, before passing it on to the Lung meridian. It has fourteen points on one side, making a total of twenty-eight if counting the bilateral points.

It starts on the inside of the big toe, runs up the inside of the leg and thigh, up to the femoral artery in the groin, to the base of the floating ribs, and up to the nipple just below the costal border.

In China it has always been said the 'the Liver governs the eyes', and this is very true, for many eye complaints can be related to liver complaints, and in addition to this, the Liver meridian has direct influence for the cure of anaemia, diabetes, neuralgia, night sweats, weakness created by cold weather, pains in the chest, abdomen and lower limbs, cystitis, arthritis in the knee, anuria, nephritis, urine troubles, muscular spasms in the chest, dyspnoea and hypertension, and leg cramps.

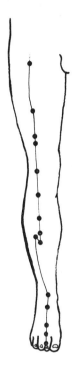

The Stomach Meridian — Fig. 25
This is another Yang meridian and it receives its Ch'i energy from the Large Intestine, and then passes it to the Spleen meridian, which we know is Yin. The Stomach meridian energy flows in a centrifugal direction, and is the second longest meridian in the body, connecting forty-five points (ninety if you count both sides), and it is the only meridian in the body where certain points are forbidden even to the acupuncturist's needle. It starts just under the eye, runs down to the side of the jawbone, then up to the top of the temples, back to the clavicle, down through the centre of the nipple, past the navel, then on to the front of the hip, thigh, leg and foot, ending in the root of the nail of the second toe.

It covers many complaints of the head (migraine, etc.), ear complaints, throat disturbances, a vast range of eye troubles, inflammation of the breast, infection of the ovaries, stomach and intestinal ailments, myositis of the lower limb, rheumatism, and arthritis in the foot and knee.

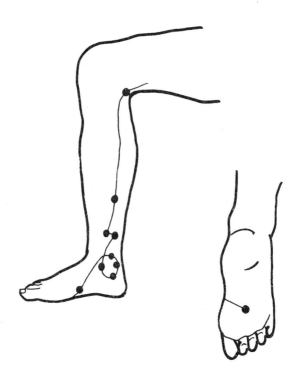

The Kidney Meridian — Fig. 26
As the Kidney meridian is under the influence of the element of water it is natural that it is Yin, and so its energy flows in a centripetal direction, and is received from the Bladder meridian, and passes on to the Heart Circulation meridian. It has a total of twenty-seven points on each side (fifty-four in all).

It starts on the ball of the foot towards the toes, carries on up the inside of the leg, first having circulated round the ankle, then runs up past the bladder, navel and breastbone to a point near the clavicle by the parastemal line.

Because of its length and the large number of meridian points, it can have great benefits for many complaints such as heart afflictions, liver affections, bladder and stomach upsets, urinary urgency, pruritis, spermatorrhoea, cystitis, eye congestions, anorexia, pulmonary emphysema, epigastric conditions, insomnia, poisoning, insufficient menses, constipation, mammitis and diabetes.

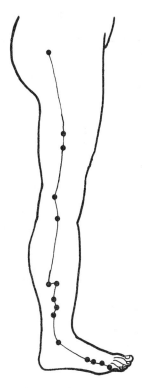

The Gall Bladder Meridian — Fig. 27
The Gall Bladder meridian is Yang and receives its Ch'i energy from
the Triple Heater meridian, in due course passing this energy on
to the Liver meridian. Being Yang, it has a centrifugal direction
of flow. It has forty-four meridian points, with a total of eighty-
eight if you count both sides.

It starts its long journey at the corner of the eye, heads towards
the lobe of the ear, and passes round the side of the head, touching
the forehead, then back over the head, down the side of the neck,
past the intercostal space, then on to the outside of the thigh, leg
and foot to the external edge of the fourth toe.

It covers all nose infections, neuralgia in different parts of the
body, leucorrhoea, inflammation of the ear, anaemia, pain and
paralysis in the face, constipation, rheumatism, urinary complaints,
cystitis, anxiety neurosis, tympanism and cancer.

The Bladder Meridian — Fig. 28
The Bladder meridian is another Yang character and receives its

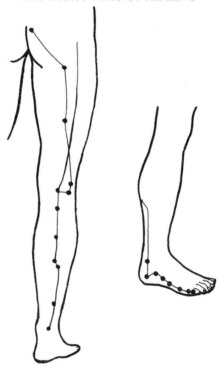

energy from the Small Intestine meridian, flowing in a centrifugal direction and then passing this energy on to the Kidney meridian. It is the longest meridian line in the body, having sixty-seven points in all, and a total of 134 if you count both sides.

It starts in the corner of the eye near the nose, goes over the head, and runs down the back in two parallel lines; it goes close to the coccyx, over the buttocks, down the back of the leg, to the rear of the outside ankle bone, then on the outside of the foot, till it reaches the external fold of the little toe.

It covers all afflictions of the heart, liver, stomach, ears, eyes and nose, as well as articular rheumatism, paralysis in many parts of the body, lung complaints, digestive complaints, mental depressions, apoplexy, constipation, stomach cancer, blenorrhagia, adenopathy, orchitis, meningitis, and troubles in the sexual organs of men and women.

So far, we have briefly described the Ch'i energy paths, which are generally referred to as the meridians of the organs, as each one is associated with an organ source which can be stimulated or tranquillized to combat specific illnesses or sickness. However, it must be appreciated that all Ch'i energy in the body will, in a truly healthy person, permeate all cells within the tissue of the complete system, and it is merely through the meridain points that we combat the symptoms of illness and influence the various organs of the body.

The Special Meridians

In addition to the twelve meridians already shown to you, there are other special energy lines, all of which have special functions, which are to act simply as containers or reservoirs to hold and regulate the use of surplus energy. So whilst the organ meridians can be likened to rivers, and the special meridians to lakes, between the lakes and the rivers there must be brooks and streams to cater for the overflow, and this smaller connection is also covered by the body, through what are called the subsidiary or extraordinary meridians.

So within the body, Ch'i energy has three main routes which it can take to help the body to keep healthy, fight disease, combat weariness in any particular part of the anatomy, and generally harmonize all the internal organs and systems into a unique and dynamic work force, these systems being:

1.   The organ meridians.
2.   The eight special meridians, or vessels.
3   The subsidiary meridians, or threads.

It is through this wonderful system of linkages that the Yin and Yang organ meridians are threaded together, and they are, in turn, connected to the vessel meridians.

With a book of this size it is impossible to cover every aspect of the meridians, but let us just show you two of the special meridians which have specific points of their own, whilst all the others do not have any particular virtues which they can call their own. These two meridians are the Conception meridian and the Governor meridian.

The Conception Meridian — Fig. 29
The Conception meridian is Yin and consists of only twenty-four points, which run directly from the gum of the lower jawbone, straight down the centre line of the body through the chest, abdomen and navel, and down to a point in front of the anus.

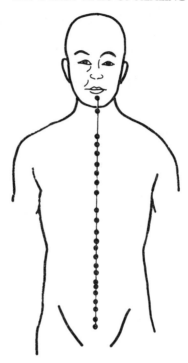

It has some important alarm points along its path which indirectly react on various organs of the body.

It has a vast influence over a huge range of illnesses. It is impossible to list them all here, but the following are a few: all diseases of the perineal area, frequent micturition, urinary diseases, vaginal discharge, irregular menses, abdominal pains, spermatorrhoea, impotence, hypertension, cerebral haemorrhage, haematuria, gastritis, cardiac pains, jaundice, insanity, palpitations, hysteria, loss of virility and energy, intestinal abscess, tongue troubles, toothache, both breasts swollen, glosillitis, swollen throat, and lung diseases.

The Governor Meridian — Fig. 30

The Governor meridian is Yang and runs from the anus to the coccyx and then up the spine, up the centre of the neck, over the head, down the centre of forehead and nose, till it arrives in the gum of the upper jawbone. It has a total of twenty-eight points.

This meridian covers a quite large range of illnesses, such as

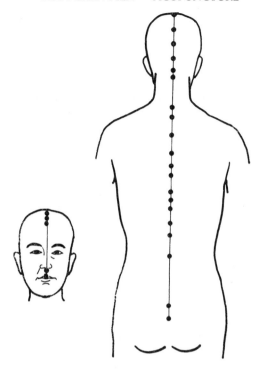

impotency, spermatorrhoea, sterility in women, haemorrhoids, rectal prolapse, retention of urine, rheumatic diseases, delirium, headaches, nervousness and insanity in children, severe fright, forgetfulness, constant weeping, hysteria, epilepsy, convulsions, painful knees, hips, back and neck, rigidity in the spine, deafness, dumbness, vaginal discharge, oedema, eyesight deterioration, diarrhoea, neurasthenia, insomnia, dyspnoea, all kinds of nasal troubles, rhinorrhoea, eclampsia, sores on the face, fainting, and red itching and pain in the corner of the eye.

The Needles and their Use
The technique of Hsia Chen Pien is normally associated with the use of needles at the various meridian points, and, as you can now fully appreciate, it is not a haphazard affair, but an exacting and very methodical science. Before commencing the treatment the practitioner must consider the complaint, the point or points to be used, the type of needle to be inserted — in terms of material, length, diameter and shape — and whether this treatment is to

be used in conjunction with other means, like heat treatment, as mentioned in Chapter 7.

As every spot or point is a nerve control centre belonging to the autonomic nervous system, the practitioner having considered all the above items will make one more test to confirm his opinion, and he does this by placing one of his fingers on the point or points to be treated. If when the point is pressed with fingertip, nothing is felt by the patient, yet when a needle is inserted into the same spot, then he gets a slight spasm of pain something like a miniature electric shock, then this indicates that the particular meridian and its associated organ are sound and functioning correctly. If, however, pain is felt when the point is pressed with the finger, and yet no pain is experienced when the needle is inserted, then that particular meridian point is malfunctioning, and it is affecting its associated organ, and so therefore it requires the necessary treatment.

So our ancient practitioner of this art had to conform to the Five Elements (Wu Hsing) before actually inserting the needle, on the following basis:
1. Complete diagnosis.
2. The meridian point or points to be treated, and the posture to be adopted, by the patient.
3. The type and length of needle to be used.
4. The direction and depth of the insertion.
5. The length of time that the needle is to be left in.

It is vitally important that the patient is placed in the right posture for the needle to be accurately placed on the appropriate point. He must also be comfortable, and in some cases the body or head may have to be propped up to keep the body firm and unmovable, yet still relaxed. Even the postures conform to the Five Elements principles:
1. Lying down on the floor on the back.
2. Lying on the stomach fully stretched out.
3. Lying on the side with the body propped in place.
4. Sitting but leaning backwards with the back supported.
5. Sitting but bending forward with the arms resting on a table.

The needle, too, must conform to the principles of the Five Elements, and as this instrument will do all the work, and obtain the necessary results, then its correct use and application play a very important part in the treatment:

1. Insertion of 90° to the surface of the skin.
2. Insertion of 45° against the flow of Ch'i.
3. Insertion of 45° with the flow of Ch'i.
4. Shallow insertion.
5. Deep insertion.

The general rules are laid down for the control of Ch'i energy in Hsia Chen Pien, and these rules are also governed by the principles of the Five Elements, and these enable every practitioner to stimulate or sedate the particular meridian point and the organ that is connected to it.

To stimulate:

1. Massage the meridian point which is to be treated, before inserting the needle.
2. Insert the needle shallowly.
3. Insert the needle slowly but in a rotary motion.
4. Insert the needle at the same angle as the flow of energy.
5. Introduce the needle as the patient exhales, and withdraw it as he inhales.

To sedate:

1. Do not massage the meridian point.
2. The needle should be inserted deeply.
3. The needle should be inserted quickly, or jabbed in, and withdrawn quickly.
4. The angle of the needle should oppose the direction of the flow of Ch'i energy.
5. The needle should be inserted as the patient inhales, and it must be withdrawn as he exhales.

Treatment is completed when the needle is withdrawn, but of course, it may be necessary for another two or three visits before the required results have been obtained. Some chronic or serious illnesses may take longer, so the course of treatment could continue for several weeks or months.

Hsia Chen Pien generally obtains quick effects, especially with those who are suffering from pain, upon which it has a responsive effect of sedation. Since 1951, records have been kept in China noting down the results of all treatments of Hsia Chen Pien, and those cases that have been successfully cured reached a remarkable total of nearly 93 per cent, which shows the effectiveness of this very ancient art. Research is still going on inside China, and in other nations of the world, and new discoveries are still being made, and all due entirely to the early teachings of the 'Sons of Reflected Light'.

Chapter 11

Tao Yin — Taoist Respiration Therapy

Respiration therapy has long been a well-known art in ancient China, and it was adopted by the Taoists, not only for its therapeutic qualities, but also because it was realized that everything within nature has to breathe to survive, so truly 'breath is life'.

So the Taoists, whose beliefs were based on very sound and rational understanding of nature and the human body, not only included respiratory exercises in their daily lives, but also experimented on a vast scale to find the true benefits and essence that air could give to the physical and spiritual sides of their lives. So it is little wonder that this dynamic medium, that helps to give and sustain life in so many things, eventually became a therapeutic system within itself, and being so closely allied to natural life, it automatically became an integral part of the Taoist way of life.

Many people believe that the respiratory art came into China in about the first century AD, when Buddhism was first introduced to the Chinese nation, but this assumption is wrong as the basic foundation of this dynamic art came with the 'Sons of Reflected Light'. However, because written records did not exist in those early days, it was not until about the sixth century BC that a mention of it was inscribed on the jade tablets, and we now know that the Taoist art of K'ai Men (Open Door), which is the Taoist yoga system of ancient China, incorporated the Yin and Yang breathing exercises within it in order to promote longevity.

There were basically twenty of these specialized respiratory exercises: eight Yin and eight Yang, and a further four which were a mixture of Yin and Yang. However, since those original exercises were devised, a further twenty exercises have been added to them, making a total of forty. All of these have a specific job to do, and that is why they are an integral part of all our Taoist arts, including Ch'ili Nung (The Way of Occlusion).

Because Tao Yin's basic principles of correct breathing are based on the foundations of Yin and Yang, and also abide by the rules of the Five Elements (Wu Hsing), this therapy has enormous potential for creating harmony between the various organs of the human body. All this is accomplished through the medium of the many different respiratory exercises, which are closely interwoven with a variety of physical movements, so that the effects and the benefits of the breathing are increased and speeded up.

Some of the exercises act as a means of sedating, some as a stimulant and a tonic, whilst others help in the activation, harnessing and cultivation of internal Ch'i energy and the external Li life force. Through the excellent health that is gained thereby, they all assist in the opening up of the whole body, enhance the functioning of the autonomic nervous system, increase the mental capacity of the brain, give greater mind control, increase perception and intuition, uplift moral standards, and give tranquillity to the mind, which in turn confers inner harmony and greater happiness. As time goes by, these exercises slowly open up the functional and control channels that feed and activate the energy, nervous and psychic centres, enabling the individual to have a deeper understanding, consciousness and awareness of the spiritual world.

Tao Yin means 'The Secret Island', and has also been known as T'u Na, which means 'Sudden Arrest', which was another way of explaining the devastating effect that the combination of breath and physical exercises has upon any illness within the human body. However, the Taoist dynamic system of breathing exercises is not a haphazard affair, for not only has it been proved over many thousands of years, but it is deep-rooted in the Taoist understanding of the principles of the universe.

The *Nei Ching* explains how methodical the ancient Taoists were in conforming to the laws of natural life. It says 'that in warm and sunny weather, when there is a full moon or it is waxing, then the flow of the breath is at its best, then a person is at the peak of their efficiency, but in colder temperatures, during the period of the new moon [no moon in the sky] or it is on the wane, then this period is Yin with very deep contractions, which will naturally affect the lungs, thereby the breathing becomes more shallow, and the person is strained and weakened'. I am writing this at the beginning of June 1983, there is no moon in the sky, and I am receiving hundreds of letters and personal callers, all suffering from hay fever or asthma; no better example of Taoist observations could be given. Because of these people, I give, in this chapter, a breathing exercise that will help those who suffer from these lung complaints.

Yin Breathing

This is very shallow breathing indeed, and it is the way that most people breathe in the Western world. It is very unhealthy and is the cause of many chest, throat and head ailments. It raises the upper chest, shoulders and collar-bone when an in-breath is taken, and it is generally known as clavicular breathing. Because it causes pressure against the diaphragm, the lungs get very little air, and this means that the blood and the body get very little benefit.

Yang Breathing

Yang breathing is very deep breathing because it concentrates on the utilization of the diaphragm. In the West it is generally referred to as diaphragmatic breathing. This way of breathing gives greater freedom to the lungs so that their absorption becomes more, creates greater elasticity in the muscles, and because of the downward pressure on the abdominal organs, which are pushed outward, it gives them an internal massage. All this is very stimulating to the lungs, which have to accept greater pressure and force, and to the lower abdomen, which is able to increase the amount of Li energy from the universe.

Yin/Yang Breathing

This type of breathing can be executed in two ways:

1. The in-breath should be as strong and take just as long as the out-breath.
2. Breathe into the chest as high as you can, then drive the air down as in diaphragmatic breathing. In the next breath, reverse this process: breathe in as low as you can, then raise the air into the lungs and chest, before breathing out.

So Tao Yin is one of the most comprehensive and dynamic exploitations of the human body, opening the way to the functions and vibrations of the psychic centres, and the control centres to and from the mind and the subconscious. All these eventually open the door to your own spirit.

It is very unfortunate that so many people in the West breathe so badly and so shallowly, using only about two-thirds of their lung capacity. Because of this there is a steady increase in the number of people with bad postures, which in turn leads to poor respiratory and circulation systems, which eventually causes many serious illnesses. All of these problems are easily curable by the simple expedient of changing the diet, and eating according to the principles of the Taoist long life therapy (Ch'ang Ming), and practising one or two specialized breathing exercises from the Tao Yin, at the right time of the day or evening.

The Taoists have proved to the world that the foundations of physical good health depend upon eating the Ch'ang Ming way, and adequate and correct breathing habits. That is one of the many reasons why so many sages and philosophers of ancient China lived to 150 or 200 years of age, because they learned to harmonize the Yin and Yang within their own bodies, through natural food and correct breathing habits at all times. They kept their flesh and bones young and supple, even in their old age, so they enjoyed the benefit of a long, healthy life.

So all those who eat, drink and breathe badly harness their bodies to sickness; those who close their minds to wisdom tie themselves to disease; whilst those who restrict or oppose the wishes of the Tao will kill their soul and so fade away.

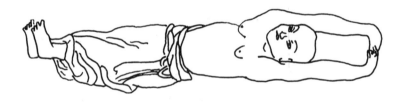

A Yin Breathing Exercise — Fig. 31
Starting position:
Lay flat on your back with your arms by your sides, and hands by your thighs.

1. Breathe in — slowly and deeply, and as you do so, raise both arms upwards in front of the body, then let the movement continue until both arms are above your head. If you can, try to rest your hands on the floor, with your fingertips touching.
2. Breathe out — very slowly, through your teeth, making a very strong, continuous hissing sound as you do so; the stronger the hiss, the more benefit will be derived. Meanwhile slowly bring your hands, in a big arc, back alongside your thighs to the starting position.

3. Repeat four more times. Those suffering from lung complaints should do this exercise in the early evening.

Benefits:
Good for asthma, hay fever, aching neck and shoulders, stiff upper arms and back.

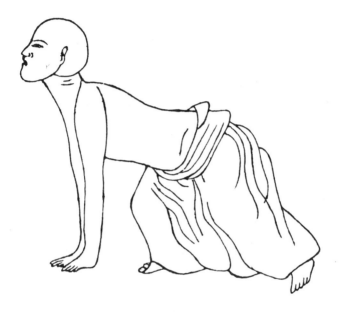

A Yang Breathing Exercise — Fig. 32
Starting position:
Stand with your feet about the width of your shoulders apart, and your hands by your sides.

1. Breathe in — deeply into the lower abdomen, and step forward with your right foot. Bend both knees as you place your hands on the floor directly under your shoulders. Your back should be straight and you should be looking straight down.
2. Breathe out — through the mouth, as you raise your back as high as you can, and bend your head downwards and try and look between your legs.
3. Breathe in — as you straighten your head and back.
4. Breathe out — as you hollow or dip your back and push your abdomen down towards the floor, at the same time, take your head back as far as you can.
5. Breathe in — as you straighten your head and back.

6. Breathe out — as you stand up and return to the starting position.
7. Repeat with the left leg forward. Now repeat the right and left posture once more. It is best if you practise this on an empty stomach.

Benefits:
Lumbago, and all back pains; gives greater strength and flexibility to the spine. Will tone the pelvic muscles, and therefore is a great aid to women in childbirth.

The importance of breathing brings about a harmony of Yin and Yang through the vibrations and pulsations that take place each time you breathe, so get into the habit of breathing deeply all the time, day in and day out, so the body can obtain the maximum benefit, as the Taoists found out many thousands of years ago.

Remember that the essence of the breath is greatest at the beginning and at the end of your life. All you have to do is fill the gap in between these two natural climaxes, so:

Learn to breathe and you will live.
Learn to breathe well — and you will retain good health.
Learn to breathe deep — and you will attain longevity.
Learn to breathe inwardly, without breathing — and you will gain spiritual immortality.

So follow this very ancient Taoist saying, and the advice that it gives — now and always.

Chapter 12

T'i Yu — Taoist Physical Culture

Ever since time immemorial the Chinese have always participated in physical movement, for personal enjoyment, for the outward expression of feeling and thought, to convey meaning without words, to keep fit and supple, to control every movement no matter how complicated a particular technique might be, to strengthen the mind, to stabilize the balance of the body, and to learn to harmonize and synchronize every unit into one beautiful and yet dynamic movement. Sometimes exercises were carried on in strictly controlled groups and accompanied by music or the beating of a drum, but more often they were practised completely alone with only nature and the universe for company. It was not uncommon for troupes of entertainers to travel the country giving displays of the complete range of their physical skills.

Not only was physical exercise used as a means of self-expression, and keeping fit, but for thousands of years, the Taoists used many aspects of it as a foundation for physiotherapy. In those early days, however, the postures, which were based on the stances, mannerisms, habits and movements of animals and birds, were rather static, and in addition the actual exercises were apt to be rather rigid, tense, hard and strenuous. So they were practised mainly by very dedicated men who had the tenacity to stick at these very vigorous work-outs.

Then, in about 1100 BC, in the Chou Dynasty, radical changes started to take place, not only in the field of physical endeavour but also in trends of thought and attitudes, and these changes were to have a dramatic effect on the future life of the Chinese nation. For all physical exercises, application and outlook took on a completely new approach, and the arts started to become softer and more pliable, and this influence reacted on the human body, which in turn began to feel the benefits.

So that the principles of this new approach should be retained by all, the Taoists formulated them according to the principles of the Five Elements (Wu Hsing):

1. Internal.
2. External.
3. Front.
4. Back.
5. Central (Tan T'ien).

These governed the human body and the development and flow of internal energy (Neichung Ch'i), or vitality power (Sheng Ch'i) and external energy (Ching Sheng Li), its direction of flow through the human body via the front and the back, and its source of activation, storage and generation (the Tan T'ien) (see Chapter 13, 'The Way of Occlusion').

Then a further five definitions were formulated to cover the use of the human body in relation to the physical movements that were to be used:

1. Head.
2. Body.
3. Arms and hands.
4. Legs and feet.
5. Balance.

Then these were again split into five, for the directions of movement had to be related to the movement or exercise, and the different types of movement needed to be specified:

1. Up and down.
2. Forward and back.
3. Sideways left and right.
4. Centrifugal.
5. Centripetal.

The Taoists were so meticulous that even these were each broken down into a further five categories, to ensure that even the smallest part was well and truly covered, and no aspect was forgotten or neglected.

So it came to be that physical exercises and movement, which at first were used primarily for self-defence and military purposes, came to be used by the general public more and more, and women and children began to participate seriously. It was then that Chinese physiotherapy began to develop hand in hand with the expansion of physical culture that now swept throughout the whole expanse of China.

The Chou Dunasty left an impressive mark in the history of Chinese internal and external development in all the creative arts, as well as in medicine and physiotherapy. It was also the era when most of the famous philosophers of China lived, such as Confucius, Mencius, Lao Tzu and Chuang Tzu, and their teachings live on to this day, for they are deeply ingrained in the lives of the Chinese, and in their upbringing and outlook.

So the Taoists according to their principles of Wu Hsing, concentrated their endeavours on the Yin and Yang balance between the internal and the external, and from this came the two arts of ultimate relationship, T'ai Chi Ch'uan (Supreme Ultimate) and K'ai Men (Open Door), which both observed the extreme law of the physical side of human life, which is 'Movement with stillness' (Yun Tung Pu Yun Tung).

However, there was one restriction which lasted over 400 years, from 206 BC until AD 220, which was during the Han Dynasty, which clamped down on all physical activities, and imposed upon the nation laws that made everyone attend educational classes, so that the standards of literature were raised. Eventually they brought in compulsory examinations which were to be sat every three years, and even when this dynasty faded out due to the many feudalistic wars which broke out in all parts of China, the civil service still retained these examinations. So whilst physical activity was harshly looked down upon during this period, it did not die out entirely, for the principles had been well and truly planted, and they proved that they were perennial, for after the Han dynasty they bloomed again, and have been in flower ever since.

So not only were the 'exterior' or 'external' arts practised with the same enthusiasm as before, but there was a greater emphasis on the practice of the softer or 'internal' arts. There came about the far deeper study of the use of internal energy as an outward force, and the utilization of the external force as an internal energy. But to attain this it meant that the physical aspects of the body had to become more pliable, more flexible and softer. So it was that T'ai Chi Ch'uan (The Supreme Ultimate), K'ai Men (Open Door), Tao Yin (Respiration Therapy) and Lien K'ang (Exercises of Peace), really came into being, and although their foundations had been laid down many thousands of years before, it was only in this era that they really became well known to the general public and their truth fully explored.

Further advancement was made through the doctrine and work of Hua T'or (AD 136-208), who is considered by many to be the father of physical culture in China, and it was he that formulated the 'five animal' method, which was based on the movements of the bear, deer, crane, tiger and monkey. This method brought out the very best of physical attainment, and at the same time he utilized the Taoist breathing exercises (Tao Yin), both of which were intended to help everyone attain the normal age of a hundred years.

The principles of his teaching were those that had been laid down by the Taoists thousands of years before, and they were based on:

1. Shen — spirit.
2. Ching — essence.
3. Chieh P'ou Shu — anatomy.
4. Chi — internal energy.
5. Li — external energy.

So in developing their understanding of the Supreme Spirit (Yuang Tati) who created the Tao (Way), the Yin and Yang, and the Five Elements (Wu Hsing), they achieved their full appreciation of the universe, and all that is within it. So the Taoists began their studies at the true beginning of life, by firstly exploring the spiritual world, then secondly, the understanding of the essence of everything. Thirdly, they completed the cycle by looking at themselves. This naturally included the whole physical make-up of their bodies, including the organs and the meridians, their health, and the energies and vitalities that make up life itself — and all Chinese Taoist health arts are based on these same fundamental principles.

T'i Yu, when used as physical therapy, should be executed without any strain or stress. It should be light and gentle at all times, comprising circular movements of the head, body, hands and arms, feet and legs. There should be no 'stopping' or 'holding' of stances or techniques, and Yang movement must be followed by Yin stillness, and then reversed. No physical strength should be used at all, for there should be complete reliance and concentration on the development and use of Ch'i initially, and eventually the harnessing, expansion and control of Li.

The upper half of the body, including arms and hands, must be followed by the lower half of the body with legs and feet, and vice versa. Motion should be slow and continuous; it should not be interrupted or halted. The mind must be at peace and in a state of tranquillity, and no thought should invade its precincts. Balance has to be maintained at all times, no matter what kind of posture or movement is executed, and the equilibrium of the Yin and Yang has to be constant.

The specialized Taoist breathing exercises (Tao Yin) must be peaceful, long and deep. Sedation and stimulation have their proper place in the arts, and one should ensure that they are used at the proper times during the day or night. Of course, whenever possible, practice should take place in the open air, and the best times are one hour after sunrise, and one hour before sunset. Remember, from a health point of view, meals should be eaten about one hour after each session, and clothing should be loose, light and comfortable.

T'ai Chi Ch'uan (The Supreme Ultimate)

Those who practise only T'ai Chi Ch'uan, which may comprise 108 to 140 movements, varying according to the school and style that is practised, are literally practising only one eighth of a complete art. In other words, they are hardly scratching the surface of this ancient art of Taoist therapeutics. For the full art comprises:

1.   The form of T'ai Chi Ch'uan.
2.   Ch'i and Li energy utilization and control.
3.   Pushing or Sticky Hands.
4.   Whirling Arms.
5.   Whirling Hands.
6.   T'ai Chi Dance.
7.   T'ai Chi Staff.
8.   T'ai Chi Sword.

T'ai Chi Ch'uan is primarily the demonstration of Yang external movements with Yin equiponderance, peace and tranquillity. The physical movements have proved themselves and their therapeutic benefits, over thousands of years, for they strengthen the limbs, increase the efficiency of the organs, tranquillize the central nervous system, improve the elasticity and texture of the skin, speed up the circulation of the blood, co-ordinate the reflex actions, benefit the lymphatic system, and help those who tend to be overweight to lose their surplus.

T'ai Chi Staff, T'ai Chi Dance and T'ai Chi Sword are normally only taught to 'advanced classes', because the physical application is more extensive and of a very high standard, where many postures have to be controlled in the air, and at times almost down to ground level. Mental control also has to be dynamic because not only are the postures vastly different, but movements are executed at a higher speed.

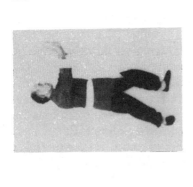
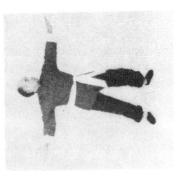
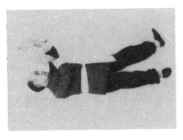
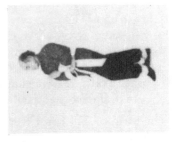
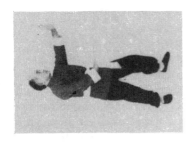
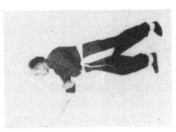
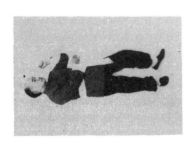
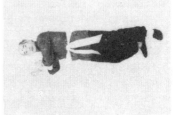

Fig. 33

Ch'i energy is also utilized at a far higher level, for not only has it to be practised inwardly, but it has also to be seen, demonstrated, and made to flow from the weapon that is held. All this comes under the heading of Ta Lu (the highway), which is the supreme road to the Supreme Ultimate.

K'ai Men (The Open Door)

This Taoist art is generally referred to as Taoist yoga in the Western world. Translated, it simply means 'Open Door' (K'ai Men), although during its long history it has also been known as Ho Ping (Unity) and Ho Hsieh (Harmony). K'ai Men (Open Door) is a very appropriate name, however, for it immediately expresses the truth, in two simple words, that it is the doorway to all the channels of the mind, body and spirit. All these, whilst retaining their own separate identity, and individual utilization, are all brought together so that they become one. That is why, in the exercises that are performed, we bring all three together in wonderful harmony, and then fully appreciate that truly at the foundations of it all, K'ai Men is the Taoist form of Ch'i Kung or energy activation, control and utilization. As we progress through this art, however, we realize even more that it doesn't stop just there, for we become aware that it is also a form of Li Kung (Energy of the Universe) supply and storage.

The Taoists certainly invented a wonderful art when they devised the art of K'ai Men, for it can be practised by children, women and men, from the very young to the very old. The exercises are soft and gentle, and you don't have to be a contortionist. From a spectator's point of view you would say it was yoga, but that's where the similarity ends, for this is all internal.

There are five 'openings' (K'ou) or 'doorways' (Men K'ou), which comprise the main sections of K'ai Men. These are spirit, mind, body, energies and healing. Naturally, there are subsections within these main sections, but every step we take within each group will certainly help us to become more aware of the depths of our own bodies, and the unity and harmony we can acquire within them.

K'ai Men goes hand in hand with T'ai Chi Ch'uan, and that is why they are both taught in a normal training session; for they are both companions that seek the same objective, although approaching it from two entirely different directions. K'ai Men has the tendency to be Yin in its external movements, but is balanced by dynamic Yang muscular changes that take place during the exercises, together with the harmonizing of the forceful flow, which is maintained under strict mental control of all the energies within the body.

As we have mentioned, K'ai Men postures and exercises are soft, light and gentle (see Fig. 34), and it is this that helps everyone to attain physical suppleness and dexterity and to reach a state of physical fitness that surprises them. And this gentleness is perfectly balanced through the Taoist understanding of the Yin and Yang.

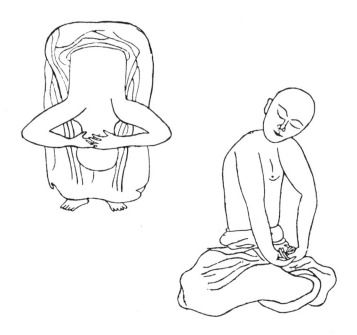

Fig. 34   Extracted from *The Book of Supple Muscles* (Ching Period).

K'ai Men also conforms to the principles of the Five Elements (Wu Hsing), which lay down the basics for this dynamic work. Naturally, first consideration is given to the spirit, and the first step is acquiring a complete understanding of the universe and how it came into being, the Tao, the Yin and Yang, and the foundation of the Five Elements in all things, as well as the consciousness and awareness of the ordained path of yourself and of all things that comprise nature.

Chapter 13

Ch'ili Nung — The Way of Occlusion

To many people in the Western world this will have no meaning whatsoever, but this is not very surprising as even the majority of Chinese do not fully appreciate its true and total depth, although some may have heard or read about little parts of it, or may have seen demonstrations of some of its usages. Even so, it is still quite a mystery to them.

The whole of this art is based on the many different types of energies or vitalities that exist or should exist within the human body if you are truly healthy. This was another of the wondrous teachings that was handed down to the Chinese by the 'Sons of Reflected Light', and humanity has received the benefits of it for thousands of years. In the Chinese health arts this is a very important factor, for part of it you were born with and learned to develop and strengthen during the stages of growing up, while other parts have to be acquired through sensible eating and drinking habits and a more cultivated way of living.

All these energies fall into five main categories, these being physical, mental, internal, external and spiritual, and they all pass through three stages of development.

Physical Development
The first section is the physical energy of our human body, which we automatically use every day of our lives, whether we are at work or at play, and this energy is being used whenever you sit down or lie down to relax, and we all accept it so naturally that very few people even give it a second thought.

Physical strength and/or brute force is not a sign of great physical energy, and as a matter of fact, in most cases this is the complete opposite, for big muscles have a tendency to retard the growth, create tensions, restrict the flow of the blood, encourage water retention, makes some organs swell in size while others contract, and all in all allow the full dynamic potential of the physical vitality to be run down or lost.

Of course, all those who are sincere and dedicated and who want to build up their physical energy, and to attain constant good health, through purification of the bloodstream, improvement of the circulation and strengthening of the organs, should first change their dietary habits. They should adopt Ch'ang Ming, the sensible eating and drinking formula, founded by the Taoists, which helps everyone to balance the Yin and Yang within themselves. Through this simple means of changing the diet, all weaknesses in the organs are eradicated, then illnesses and sickness become just a distant memory, and you will then attain the perfect good health that is the natural heritage of every human being. In other words, physical health perfection that was once a dream now becomes true reality.

Once you attain the true health of your own body, so that not even a common cold will ever enter your life again, then your physical energy will have the strength to fight all bacteria and viruses that happen to come your way, and you will be able to grow old in years, yet retain the vitality of your youth in conjunction with excellent physical good health.

Mental Development

Mental energy (Chingshen) is also used in a great variety of ways, such as through the normal channels of thinking, for the discipline and control of the movements of the limbs, counteracting the emotional drain on our lives and the replacement of vitalities imposed by stress or strain. It is also used at a very high level under all conditions of everyday life — playing, working, driving, etc., as well as being used in directions of which you are not always aware, such as your sense of taste, intuition, sensory perception, hypersensitivity, and of course, all the various aspects of Mo Kung (Taoist Wand) and Mo Hsiang (Taoist meditation), both of which are vast fields in themselves.

Then of course the mental energy is used to control, harness, channel and develop all other vitalities within the human body, and not only during the day when the body is active, but also at night when you are asleep. So you will appreciate that complete and utter relaxation of the mind, body and spirit is absolutely essential for the retention of good health, but it is also a major key to our personal life, for when we relax completely the channels within the body and the head can be thrown wide open to allow the free flow of vitality. They can also be closed by your own will and control, to ensure that such energies are not wasted unnecessarily, and therefore you can learn how to store them until the time comes when they are wanted for an essential purpose. That is why it is important for the attainment and the reinforcement of good health, and is of primary importance to positive advancement to even further goals in the mental and spiritual aspects of your life.

Let this be your aim in life, to get a truly healthy body (and not necessarily a physically fit body), by adhering to the Ch'ang Ming way of eating and drinking, so that you will be able to gain, retain, store and recharge your mental energy, then you will be able to increase the power of your internal energy, and then go on to the next step, which is that of developing the external field of force as well. Whilst these things might all seem to be separate, which indeed they are — in their own particular spheres of operation, it is essential that they can also be harmonized, under your mental control, so that they can eventually become one entity.

The next sections are the major fields of Ch'ili Nung. Unfortunately most people allow them to go to waste, or they allow their little-used — yet vital — physical and mental energies to be depleted to such low levels that they are unable to gain control of them. Thus they are frittered away and lost for ever. So the average person will never know the joy and happiness that these vitalities can bring, nor really appreciate how important they are to their own physical, mental and spiritual lives.

Internal Energy

The whole health of the human body is based on 'internal energy' (Neichung Ch'i), more commonly known as the 'vitality power' (Sheng Chi, or simply Ch'i) and it is one of the most important aspects of the 'Eight Strands of the Brocade' (Pa Chin Hsien). Its force is truly dynamic, its utilization is fantastic, and its benefit to a person's good health is beyond normal comprehension. Everyone practising our Taoist arts endeavours to develop, activate and cultivate Ch'i, for not only is it an important factor in the good health of the body and mind, but it also has spiritual ramifications as well.

The 'Supreme Spirit' (Yuhuang Tati) has created some wonderful things in this world, and Sheng Chi is one of them, but to try and explain it to you in simple terminology, and still give you a real understanding of what it is all about, is difficult to say the least. The Taoists of China have benefited from their awareness and understanding of it for many thousands of years, and have attained very long lives, some of them being reputed to have lived to be 150 or 200 years of age.

It is the natural internal power of the human body, and it is a far greater force than sheer physical brute strength can ever be, and what is more amazing is the fact that you were born with it, but over the years you have allowed its power to decline or become dormant within your own body. In its own way it helps to fight germs and bacteria within the body, and so effectively that you will find that colds and flu will not affect you, and your general health will improve beyond your wildest dreams.

We know what it is, how it can be stored, how it can be controlled, activated and cultivated, and where it emanates from, and we also know the effects that it has on the health of our own bodies. We also know that we can heal others with it too, and that it can be expressed from the human body over many hundreds of yards. It is an intangible force, invisible to the eyes, cannot be heard, and it has no smell, and whilst it consists of an immaterial substance, yet it is very materialistic. It is substantial yet enormously insubstantial, it is unresisting yet at the same time it can be pliability itself. It has no weight at all yet it cannot be lifted, it is soft and gentle like a morning breeze and yet it can be as hard as iron. It can be sensed, however, if your sensory perception is strong enough or has been sufficiently trained to recognize the symptoms. It is life and the centre of your own life, for all humanity is born with it. It came into being when you were in your mother's uterus, and it will only leave you when you take in your last breath.

Your Ch'i is always with you, but unfortunately when you were about five or six years of age you started to use your physical and muscular strength more and more and your Ch'i less and less. In some people it lies almost dormant through poor health and lack of use. Therefore it has to be revived and reactivated, and initially there are a few obstacles that have to be overcome, but once having coerced your Ch'i to flow, then you can spend time in cultivating it day by day, so that it becomes stronger and stronger as each day goes by. Everything will depend on your own personal dedication, for there are no short cuts, and everyone has to go through all the stages, one by one, before the absolute ultimate can be obtained. Then, and only then, will you have obtained the dynamic benefits of constant good health, a tranquil mind, peace and happiness, and longevity. There are many records of the Taoists of China living to very ripe old ages, all in perfect health and with all their mental faculties working as efficiently as when they were much younger. But of course, with the greater maturity of age, they had the greater understanding, appreciation, experience and wisdom that only time can bring, with the added benefits of the dynamic energies that guaranteed them greater spiritual outlook and strength.

First Stage
The first principle involved in gaining Internal Power (Ch'i) is to relax in mind, body and spirit, but we know that true relaxation is one of the hardest objectives to achieve. It is no good going to the nearest armchair and flopping into it, for this type of relaxing is merely giving up all your physical energies, and thereby your muscles, tendons, tissues and mind become slack and lazy. In our Taoist arts we use the periods when the body should be relaxed to store energy, so that we always have the power available whenever we require to use it. There are no prescribed periods when you should relax, but you must be able to adjust yourself so that you can learn to do it whenever you wish, whether you are at work or at play, walking or sitting down. So you may fully appreciate that one of the first steps on this upward path, is to throw the whole of your physical and mental spheres wide open, so that there is not the slightest obstruction internally, thereby there is not the slightest stress or strain. Going strictly on to the Ch'ang Ming diet will help you enormously to attain this goal.

The next stop in this first phase is to build up the natural energy of the body. Liken yourself to a storage heater: when it is working it is pumping heat out into the room, but when it is not doing so during the off-peak period, then it stores the heat within itself to be used at a later time. This is exactly the same principle on which your Ch'i works, for when we give ourselves time to relax, then we use that period to conserve and store further energy, and as internal power or Ch'i is heat, then you will readily understand the relationship that exists.

However, we do need something to speed up the process of making more energy, at the same time ensuring that we have adequate storage. So at this stage, you should not only eat the Taoist Ch'ang Ming way but should also incorporate into your daily life the various Taoist breathing exercises which will help in the process of relaxing and will also aid the generation of more heat so that more energy can be produced and a greater capacity made available to be stored.

Second Stage

This stage is known to us as the 'Propelled Movement' (T'uichin Yuntung) period, when the trainee will start to learn how to direct the Ch'i from the lower abdomen to various parts of the body at will. If you turn on a tap or valve you know that you can open the channel so that the water will start to flow down the pipe, without having to activate the pipe, or you could, for instance, switch on an electrical connection and know that as soon as you do so, the electricity will flow along the wires, without you having to move the wires in the process. Your bones, muscles and tissues become the pipes and the wires, and inside them are the channels along which the energy of your body will flow, and they will carry your Ch'i to any part of the body, without any physical movement on your part. In other words, you do not need a single ounce of physical or muscular strength to help the flow of your internal energy.

Again in this stage there are specialized Taoist breathing exercises that are incorporated to give an added stimulus to the flow and an aid to the mental control over directional diversions, and they also assist in locking the Ch'i at specific points in the functional and control channels of the body, as well as within the psychic centres that are themselves central emanation points.

There can be no time limit set for the length of this stage, as it is entirely dependent upon the individual's capacity for personal dedication, strength and attitude of mind, and depth and control of relaxation, as well as on overall bodily health, the amount of heat generation, the quality and quantity of the storage centres, and the ability to control and fully utilize the energy flow.

The golden rules of this stage are:

1. Gain complete mastery of yourself.
2. Attain complete and utter relaxation of the mind, body and spirit.
3. Get the feel of generating this internal energy and heat.
4. Learn how to hold and store it carefully.
5. Learn how to control and direct it to any part of the human anatomy where it might be needed.

Third Stage

This is the most advanced stage of internal power, but it is within the reach of everyone providing they are willing to allow themselves time to reach it. If you have the mental aptitude and constant dedication you could reach it in five or six years, or it could take you fifty years, and there again, there are many who never reach it at all. It all depends entirely upon your own personal dedication.

Ch'i, as we have already mentioned, is a form of heat, and it can be propelled to any part of the body at will. Your abdomen (Tan T'ien), where the Ch'i energy is stored has only a very limited capacity, and therefore, sooner or later, it will begin to overflow. This is the initial aim, to be able to make so much vitality that it will overflow more and more. A further Taoist breathing exercise is introduced at this point to increase the overflowing action, and then to try and ensure that this overflow is maintained on a more permanent basis, and in so doing the heat potential is also boosted, and the health of the body becomes so good that even the common cold or a headache becomes a memory of the past. We in the Taoist arts have ways and means of proving the amount of flow and the degree of its force, and at various intervals in time each practitioner can gauge his own rate of progression through these simple tests.

At first, internal power will fall from the abdomen (Tan T'ien) into the lower extremities of the pelvis (Ku P'an) and as the action continues, the force of energy is driven up the spine, over the top of the head, through the control channels which are operated by the mind, and then down the front of the body through the functional channels, and finally back to the abdomen. Whilst making this journey, the overflow action will also fill the muscles, tendons and sinews of the body, giving them added strength, greater flexibility and more pliability. However, everything depends on good eating habits such as those of Ch'ang Ming. If bad eating habits are normal (as in most Western families) then restrictions and deep contractions hamper or stop the flow of energy to various parts of the body, and then sickness prevails.

The bones of the body are a different proposition for they are all sealed units, which makes the penetration of inner power very difficult and the process of intake very much slower. It can and does penetrate to the innermost part of every bone, however, providing the Ch'i energy is strong, by a process which is known as osmosis.

Without becoming too technical, osmosis can be explained as follows. As the muscles, tendons and tissues of the body become heated through the flow of Ch'i energy, that heat is passed automatically to the outside surface of the bone, because they are all in very close proximity to one another. Then slowly the bone itself becomes heated all the way through, and this heat, in turn, is transmitted to the marrow.

The bone and marrow become tempered through a sweating action that takes place in the process. This tempering will make their texture so hard and resilient that they become like steel, and yet, in the same process, they both become more supple than ever before. That is why amongst the Taoists bone marrow diseases are unheard of, and that is another reason why the development of Ch'i is encouraged by everyone who practises our arts.

Once this supreme unification has taken place, then you will have reached the ultimate level of mastery and control of your own internal power (Sheng Chi); you will have reached the stage of rejuvenation; and you will be able to ward off all diseases, and also prolong the span of your own life.

It is not known how old the 'Sons of Reflected Light' lived to be, but my master said that he was told that it was believed to be hundreds of years of age. So why not let this be your way of life too, for not only will you be more evenly tempered, for all tensions will be taken out of your life, but you will be much happier, for nothing will upset your daily life. You will also attain constant good health, and extend your lifespan in so doing.

External Energy

This source of energy is vital to our own personal lives. It is known as 'macrocosmic energy' (Ching Sheng Li) and it is akin to the ether that supports the planets of the universe. We know that it does exist even though it cannot be seen. It is billions of years older than the world we live in, yet it is extremely young, and it became a part of your life before you left your mother's womb. This energy comes down from the heavens, passes through all Yang things with a centripetal motion, and then enters the earth, where it accumulates further vitality. It then returns from whence it came, but in doing so it passes upwards through all Yin things, in a centrifugal circular action.

Macrocosmic energy is everywhere, and it passes through you constantly. Even as you sit reading this, this energy is passing through you. If you can learn to harness it, store it, control it and utilize it, then you can reach the realms of immortality as the Taoists learned to do many thousands of years ago. They also learned to use it for the purpose of healing others, and it is still being used for this purpose today. It is more dynamic than internal energy

(Sheng Chi) and it can also be controlled through the mind. However, in this case, it is projected through the pineal gland, which the Taoists call the Golden Gate (Chin Men), and it is the first step towards the Supreme Ultimate (Tsui Kao Tsuihou).

It gives life and vitality to all plants, for without it they would droop and die, and our own life pattern is dependent on it as well. In our Taoist arts we have known for over 4,000 years that cancer is due to very low internal and external energy, and all that is necessary is to build up these two energies in a person and cancer is eliminated. So work and strive for truly good health by eating the Ch'ang Ming way, and aim to obtain the ultimate goal yourself by developing your energies, and life will take on a new meaning for you.

Healing

Healing, unlike acupuncture, does not require special instruments, and we don't need any special herbs either; all we need is personal good health, strong energies, understanding of the Yin and Yang, and a good understanding of the meridian channels in the body. Remember, too, that we can practise healing on ourselves as well as on other people, although if you are truly eating the Ch'ang Ming way then you will never be ill, unless you break the dietary rules, in which case your stomach will let you know very quickly.

Vibration Healing

This is accomplished in two entirely different ways. The first is either created by the patient himself or can be passed on by the helper through the vibration of a specific sound which will have a Yin or Yang effect on an organ or organs of the body. The second alternative is through the vibration of Ch'i down a specific meridian channel of the body, which again will have its benefits on a specific area or organ. It was only the positive and very deep understanding of the Yin and Yang, that enabled the ancient Taoists to explore the human body to such great depths.

Ch'i and Li Healing

As you will guess, these utilize both our internal and external energies for healing purposes, and both are used on a Yin and Yang basis, depending on the cause of illness. Both can be performed either by the patient himself or by a helper. With Ch'i healing it is important to have a good knowledge of the meridian channels, so that these can be fully utilized during a healing session. Each organ has its own meridian, which begins or ends at a certain finger or toe, so if we want to treat a lung complaint, then we place one hand on the lung and the other hand on the outside edge of the thumbnail. In the West this would probably be called palm healing. Li healing is very similar except that we must accept an adequate supply of Li energy, which means we must be very healthy, and on Ch'ang Ming preferably, through one hand whilst the other hand rests on the sick organ. The angle of the free hand will depend on whether you are male or female, in other words, Yin or Yang, and on the sex of the patient. Simple adaptations can then be made.

Meditation

There are many ways of meditating in Taoism, and, whilst these can be listed as twenty basic and separate paths, they are divided into many subsections, which makes the field of Taoist meditation very large indeed. Yet, because of the balance of Yin and Yang, it is highly contractive as well as being enormously expansive, and this therefore allows us to explore deep within ourselves and others, and to travel all over our own world, as well as transcending to the astral plane, the celestial sphere, and even the heavenly orbit.

If you reach the stage when you can meditate fully whenever you wish, and in any of the sections that you choose, then you may progress even further by exploring how to meditate with your eyes open. We call this 'visual transportation' (Shih Li Yun Shu). Then there is a further stage, which is called 'spiritual transportation' (Ching Shen Yun Shu). Both are very advanced stages of Taoist meditation, and you need a very good teacher to help you through the various stages, but here are a few points that are worth remembering:

1. Put your tongue into the roof of the mouth.
2. Breathe in and out of the nostrils only.
3. Breathe the Yang way for energy activation.
4. Eradicate all rising thoughts and cleanse the mind.
5. Erase all feelings, sounds and smells from your senses.
6. Morning and evening are the best times for meditating.
7. The minimum requirement is one meditation per day.
8. The best time is in the morning.
9. Start by meditating for fifteen minutes, then slowly work up to one hour.
10. Each morning, massage the abdomen before getting out of bed, and before meditating, practise a few deep breaths, then go to the toilet. You are now ready to start.

Appendix

The International Taoist Society

The Lee Family

The history of the Taoist arts within the Lee family goes back well over 3,000 years. At that time, the family lived in the town of Wei Hei Wei, a fishing port approximately 200 miles from Peking. The Lee family practised the Taoist arts continuously, but no one knows how they originally came into the family possession. Not only did they possess these priceless arts, they also managed to hand them down from generation to generation for all these years.

To keep the arts so complete and in their original state was no mean feat and it means that all the members of the family had to have very deep and sincere dedication throughout the ages. History alone will tell us how hard the study of all these arts was. This applies especially to the art of T'i Yu (physical culture), which in its original state was extremely hard and rigid, although with changes in attitude and understanding it eventually softened into a very gentle form of calisthenics.

Chan Kam Lee

Chan Kam Lee was the last in line of the Lee family, and as he was an importer and exporter of precious and semi-precious stones, he travelled thousands of miles promoting his business, which was mainly between Hong Kong, Japan, Singapore and England. After he had built up a stable business he finally set up his main office in London, and from there he did most of his trade.

After a while Chan Kam Lee began to get restless, and he sought an outlet for his physical, mental and spiritual needs. As a result, he established a small and select class in a schoolroom in Red Lion Square, near Holborn, in Central London, teaching and practising his Chinese Taoist arts. He catered only for his own personal friends and their sons, so the total number of his students was very small, and at the most there were only a dozen people attending. All of them were in business and travelled quite a lot, so the average attendance at any one time was only in the region of six people. However, this did not deter Chan Lee for he was able to keep up his own practice as well, which was the main objective in the first place, so he was very happy.

Chee Soo

Chee Soo was born of a Chinese father and an English mother, and as they died when he was only a very young child, he was brought up in a Dr Barnardo's home, which was and still is a charitable orphanage. He started his first job, as a page-boy in a nursing home in Earls Court, West London, and in his spare time he used to go to Hyde Park to enjoy the fresh air, watch the horse riders exercising their animals, and to play with his ball.

However, something happened that was to alter the whole course of his future life. One Sunday afternoon, he went to the park to play with his ball, when suddenly it bounced rather erratically, and accidentally hit the back of an elderly gentleman who was sitting on a park bench. Having recovered his ball, he went up to the gentleman to offer his apologies, only to see that the man was also Chinese. As it was a very rare thing to see another Chinese in London in those days, they began to talk together, and even arranged to meet again. So the two began to meet fairly regularly — whenever the opportunity and the weather permitted, and a very strong friendship developed between Chee Soo and the gentleman, who was Chan Kam Lee.

In the summer of 1934, Chee Soo was invited to Chan Lee's class, and that was the beginning of the training that he has maintained ever since, and it was surely the ordained way of the *Tao* that enabled Chee Soo to start his learning of the vast range of the Taoist martial, philosophical, healing and cultural arts in this way. It gave great happiness to Chan Lee for he had no family of his own, and as he earnestly desired to keep the Taoist arts alive, he adopted Chee Soo as a nephew, and taught him the arts whenever his work and time permitted. For Chee Soo it meant that the he had someone on whom he could rely, and to advise him, and teach him the fundamentals of the Taoist philosophical attitude to life and all that it meant.

In 1939 the Second World War broke out, and Chee Soo did his share of fighting as a Tank Commander in the Second Battalion of the Royal Tank Corps, in France, in North Africa — where he won the Military Medal, and in Burma where, after a hectic battle, he was finally taken prisoner by the Japanese. He went through many periods of beatings, torture, starvation and very hard work as a member of a working party in the mountains between India and Burma. Finally, three years later, as the Japanese started to retreat from the advancing Allies, he managed to escape into the Shan Mountains of West Burma and made his way over very rugged terrain and through many jungles, till finally one month afterwards he was able to make contact with the Allies again. Three months after recuperation and treatment (for he then weighed only 84 lbs), he was flown back to England, where he was able to enjoy a long leave with his wife. After that, he was discharged from the forces and took a course in book-keeping, stock control, commercial history and sales promotion.

He managed to make contact with Chan Lee again after the war was finished, and the class in Holborn was restarted. In 1950, Chee Soo, with Chan Lee's permission, formed his own class in Manor Road School, West Ham, East London.

The Formation of the International Taoist Society

This society was formed on the foundations that were originally laid down by Professor Chan Kam Lee to cater for the interest that was beginning to be aroused, and because other members started to form their own classes and clubs, and it was felt that the formation of an association would help to bind all practitioners together.

In the winter of 1953-4, Chan Lee died, off the coast of China, near Canton, when the ship that he was travelling in sank in a severe storm, and so Chee Soo was asked to take over the leadership of the Association. However, in deference to the memory of Chan Lee, Chee Soo declined to accept any title within the Association at that particular time. By 1959, groups and clubs were being formed all over the world, and they were all asking for leadership. For this reason, Chee Soo decided to accept the post of President of the Association. Since then the Association has grown from strength to strength in the British Isles, Australia, South Africa, France, Germany Holland, Mauritius and New Zealand.

Only the Taoist arts of the 'Eight Strands of the Brocade' are taught within this association and these comprise:

Ch'ang Ming (Taoist long life health diet therapy).
Ts'ao Yao (Taoist herbal therapy).

Anmo (Taoist massage).
Tao Yin (Taoist respiration therapy).
Tien Chen (Taoist acupressure — spot pressing).
T'i Yu (physical culture).
Chen Tuan (Taoist diagnosis techniques).
Ch'ili Nung (The Way of Occlusion).

There are two other associations which are affiliated to our society:

The Chinese Cultural Arts Association, who teach:

T'ai Chi Ch'uan (the Supreme Ultimate).
K'ai Men (Taoist yoga or the Taoist form of Ch'i Kung).
I Fu Shou (Sticky Hands).
Li Kung (Taoist development of Li energy).
Mo Kun (Taoist wand for Li energy control).
Mo Hsiang (Taoist meditation).

also T'ai Chi dance, Tai Chi stick and T'ai Chi sword.

The International Wu Shu Association, who teach:

Feng Shou ('Hand of the Wind' Kungfu, very soft, very gentle,
    and very fast, suitable for women and men of all ages).
Chi Shu (a Taoist form of Aikido).

and all other Taoist self-defence arts, including those involving
weapons.

Coaching
Since taking over as President, Chee Soo has set up the Area
Coaching Centres, with the object of training serious and dedicated
people to become qualified instructors and teachers, and also to
ensure that the high standards of physical and mental application
are maintained everywhere, and only the Taoist arts are taught.
This has proved extremely successful and centres now exist in many
parts of the country, and a wonderful standard of skill, knowledge,
technique and energy are prominent at all levels. Periodic
examinations are held every year, and the Association's Coaching
Certificates and Awards are recognized throughout the world.

Needless to say, all our associations strictly maintain the
traditions and rules that were laid down by Profesor Chan Kam
Lee and his family; and our President, Professor Chee Soo, who
naturally, is also a Taoist, has dedicated his whole life in serving
and helping others whenever he can.

Anyone interested in the true Taoist arts of ancient China, can join their local classes or clubs, and can also attend the student coaching classes, which are held regularly throughout the British Isles and in Europe. If you wish to know the nearest class or club or coaching centre to your home, don't hesitate to write to us, and we will do all we can to help. Details can be obtained from:

Mrs M. Perkin
Honorary Secretary
426 Charter Avenue
Canley
Coventry CV4 8BD
West Midlands
England

Index